The Complete Book
of Stretching

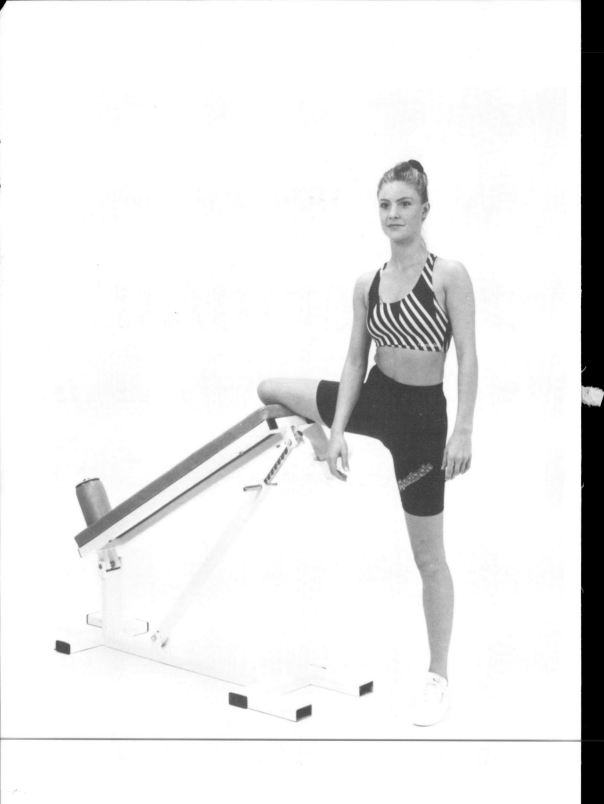

The Complete Book of
STRETCHING

TONY
LYCHOLAT

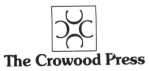

The Crowood Press

First published in 1990 by
The Crowood Press
Ramsbury, Marlborough
Wiltshire SN8 2HR

New edition 1995
This impression 1998

British Library Cataloguing in Publication Data

A catalogue record for this book is available from the British Library.

ISBN 1 85223 917 4

Typesetting by Butler and Tanner Ltd, Frome and London
Printed and bound in Great Britain by J. W. Arrowsmith Ltd, Bristol

Contents

Acknowledgements

As ever, thanks to everyone who helped in the writing and production of this book, especially Anne-Marie O'Keefe for being such an excellent model and Roy Wooding for taking such good photographs. Reebok (UK) Ltd were also kind enough to supply the clothing and footwear which features in the majority of the illustrations and their support is appreciated. Many people also helped indirectly in arriving at the final content of this book, and they too must be thanked. So, thanks to all those teachers, instructors and students who have either shown me an exercise, or who have taught me something by allowing me to teach them.

1 The Benefits of Stretching

More and more athletes, sportsmen and women, recreational exercisers and members of the general public seem to be finding time to stretch. Once the province of the yogi or the circus contortionist, stretching exercises are now seen by many as an integral part of all exercise and training sessions and as an aid to many situations encountered in everyday life. If you do not regularly engage in stretching exercises, or if you do but are not sure of the benefit of your stretches, this chapter, dealing with the considerable advantages of regular stretching should leave you utterly convinced of the role of stretching with regard to improving both your sports performance and your general health and well-being.

STRETCHING AND THE SPORTS PERFORMER

Whilst it is true to say that there are many highly successful sports performers who do not engage in regular stretching exercises, such sportsmen and women are becoming the exception rather than the rule.

Stretching exercises offer many advantages to the sports performer in a wide variety of ways. Initially, as part of the warming-up process, when all sports performers are preparing their bodies for the more strenuous, often all-out activity which is about to follow, a period of preparatory stretches will ensure that all muscles, joints and limbs have been carefully taken throughout their full range of movement. Having done this as part of the warm-up phase, the body is then not 'shocked' when it is asked to go through those ranges of movement during the competitive physical activity or sport itself. Consequently, the risk of injuring muscles, joints and joint structures such as ligaments, is much less if the performer warms up and stretches appropriately prior to engaging in more strenuous physical exercise.

Stretching exercises, if correctly executed and if they follow a progressive pattern, will also lead to an increase in an individual's normal range of movement. In other words, regular, appropriate stretching will lead to an increase in a person's flexibility. This is of benefit to sports performers, since all other things being equal, the greater the range of movement that a person has throughout his or her joints, the greater the amount of force that he or she can apply to the ground, to water, to objects and to implements. For example, if you wish to run fast, what ultimately determines your speed is how quickly your legs go round (your cadence), and how much ground you cover with each stride. Sprinters, for example, are characterised by having a naturally fast cadence, and a long stride length. It is the combination of these two factors which leads to the phenomenal speed which world-class sprinters exhibit. The training of sprinters ensures that not only can they exert high forces with their muscles, but they can exert those forces throughout as full a range of movement as possible – and the longer they can apply force, the more total force is exerted, and generally speaking, the more impressive the performance.

The same is true of applying force to water, as in swimming, where élite swimmers will move their hands and arms in elaborate curves to apply as much force as possible to the water, hence moving faster and more efficiently. For further illustration of this point, consider kicking a football, or throwing an implement like a discus or javelin. To kick a ball a long way, does your leg move through a wide arc, or a short one? The wider the arc of the kick, the more the foot at the end of the leg accelerates, imparting the highest possible force to the football, which if struck to follow the right trajectory, will travel the greatest possible distance.

The techniques of throwing implements like the javelin or discus have also evolved largely to allow the thrower to exert force for as long as possible, throughout as full a range of movement as possible, to the object to be launched. Examples such as these hopefully serve to indicate that the greater the range of movement a performer has, the greater his or her potential for applying force – accepting of course that the competitor in question has the necessary ability to generate force!

Stretching exercises, aimed at developing flexibility or range of movement, are also of tremendous value to sports performers in helping them to correct certain deficiencies in technique. As most people will have experienced, the most successful performers are invariably those who have the best technique. This is because a highly skilled practitioner expends the right amount of energy in the right direction, unlike the dissipated efforts of the less highly skilled individual. In some instances incorrect technique may be a problem because there is a range of movement imbalance at certain joints. Excessively tight hamstring muscles may, for example, limit how effectively individuals can move their legs throughout the range of movements required for sprinting. Solving this problem by performing the appropriate stretching exercises will obviously improve the execution of the necessary movements and improve the individual's sprinting technique in general. It is also worth noting that excessively tight muscles may also predispose a sports performer to injury. Using the hamstring muscles again as an example, note the instance of injury

so often seen to occur to these muscles in sprinters who neglect to warm up and stretch appropriately.

Sports performers – and indeed many over-enthusiastic recreational exercisers – will also be familiar with the rather unpleasant sensations of delayed onset muscle soreness (DOMS). This is soreness and stiffness which can be extremely acute and which is invariably brought about through extremely vigorous or unaccustomed exercise or strenuous physical activity. Unlike other forms of less severe soreness associated with exercise, DOMS does not appear until at least a whole day (more usually two) after the activity in question.

Whilst there is virtually no scientific evidence at the moment to support the anecdotal evidence that stretching exercises can prevent DOMS from occurring, or that stretching helps to alleviate DOMS when it does occur, many athletes will argue that stretching is very useful as far as DOMS is concerned. To prevent DOMS, according to some sportsmen and women, carry out a full, progressive stretching routine at the end of your work-out or training session. To alleviate the sensations of DOMS, so the theory goes, warm the affected muscles thoroughly and then engage in light stretching.

STRETCHING FOR EVERYBODY

Obviously, much of what has been said with reference to the sports performer is also of value to the recreational exerciser. Certainly if you are exercising just for the health and fitness benefits it still makes good sense to structure your exercise session so that it contains a thorough warm-up, including preparatory stretching, and a thorough warm-down, including progressive, developmental stretching designed to increase your range of movement. It is also worth bearing in mind that flexibility is one of the five accepted health-related components of physical fitness (along with muscular strength, muscular endurance, cardio-respiratory endurance and body composition). These components of physical fitness are deemed 'health-related', precisely because an improvement in any or all of them will lead to improvements in health and well-being.

The health aspects of improved range of movement, brought about through regular progressive stretching are perhaps only fully appreciated when normal range is lost or suspended for a while because of illness or injury. Only when a limb is immobilised (in a cast, for example) or when we watch an arthritic person struggling to carry out a simple movement task do we fully realise the importance of having a free and easy range of movement throughout all our joints.

Being flexible enables us to reach, bend, twist and turn with ease, making everyday tasks involving movement that much more straightforward and simple to execute. It is also noticeable that an appropriate balance of flexibility and strength in all the major muscle groups enables the best possible posture to be maintained. This point is very important, since having the right posture, whether standing, sitting, driving or performing any activity is necessary if you are to perform that activity easily and avoid injury. It is perhaps obvious that lifting heavy objects with poor posture can lead to all kinds of injuries to muscles and joints. However, it invariably escapes most peoples' notice that sitting badly for long periods is equally injurious, if not more so, since anatomical changes associated with poor sitting and standing postures tend to be more insidious in nature, creeping up on the individual and only making themselves apparent when more major problems have occurred.

Take the many reported instances of neck, back and shoulder injuries associated with poor sitting positions in front of a VDU screen as an example – an increasingly common problem in large companies. With bad sitting posture many people effectively end up slouching in front of their screens and keyboards, placing muscles and joints in very odd positions. As the positions are held and repeated on a regular, daily basis, some muscles become habitually shortened whilst others become habitually lengthened. The new positions the body finds itself in may also lead to pressure being exerted upon other structures within the body, such as blood vessels, nerves and organs. It is these pressures on muscles, joints, nerves, blood vessels and organs that cause so many posture-related ailments, from aching limbs and joints to headaches, circulatory disorders and breathing problems. Whilst most people can easily appreciate how sitting badly can cause the health problems mentioned, what might be less obvious is the fact that standing and moving badly are equally problematical.

Whilst appropriate stretching may not solve all postural problems, certain exercises, if repeated often enough can help to get the body back into normal alignment, enabling it to function correctly. Such postural exercises also have the added advantage of improving your shape, since good posture instantly improves your appearance. Clearly, the benefits of regular stretching are profound, whoever you are and whatever your reason for stretching. As will also be seen in Chapter 2, it does not matter how old you are either, since stretching exercises can be carried out by all age groups with great success. However, before you begin any stretching programme it is necessary to understand more about the nature of movement at joints, and movement limitations in order to make certain that the stretches you intend to carry out are safe and appropriate for you. It is also a good idea to establish your current range of movement. These points are dealt with in the next chapter.

2 Normal Ranges of Movement

People who can perform the splits have a greater than normal range of movement, and can often perform this impressive feat because of a naturally more favourable joint and muscle arrangement than that which exists in the average person. Consequently, aspiring to perform the splits, or attempting other similar extreme limb positions is invariably hazardous for most people not in the possession of the necessary joint laxity. It is always worth bearing this point in mind if you have visions of becoming extremely flexible as a result of your stretching programme. For, as with other forms of exercise and training, the results you are likely to achieve from your training programme will be ultimately determined by your genetic make-up, as well as by the amount of appropriate work you put in.

Naturally enough, careful consideration of your own basic anatomy, plus an understanding of how your muscles and joints work will also enable you to continually ensure that every stretch position you attempt is safe and will lead to an increase in your range of movement, and not to injury. So before launching into any stretch exercise, ask yourself: is this movement anatomically possible for me? To help you answer this question, this chapter explains just how movement occurs at joints.

UNDERSTANDING MOVEMENT

All movements in the body occur at what are known as joints. A joint is simply a meeting place between bone and bone, or cartilage and bone. The amount of movement which is possible at a joint initially depends upon how the joint in question is put together. Some bones, for example, are held together by strong, fibrous connective tissue. A typical example of such a fibrous joint are the joints, or sutures, between the bones of the cranium. Fibrous joints allow no movement. Other bones are held together by cartilaginous connective tissue. Cartilaginous joints, such as those between successive vertebrae in the spine, allow limited movement. (The fact that there is such a wide range of movement of the spinal column in general reflects the summation of all the small movements possible between the vertebrae.) The most freely moveable joints of all are known as synovial joints (*see Fig 1*). In a synovial joint

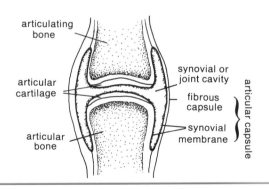

Fig 1   A typical synovial joint showing the main features.

there is a space between the opposing bones and the ends of the bones are enclosed in a tough connective sheath known as the synovial (or joint) capsule. The inner surface of the synovial capsule is known as the synovial membrane which secretes a fluid known as synovial fluid – this nourishes and lubricates the joint structures within the capsule. Synovial joints also feature other structures, such as ligaments, which are placed in such a position around the joint so as to afford considerable strength to the joint, effectively preventing unwanted movement in certain directions. Discs of cartilage may also be found in some synovial joints to allow independent movement of the separate bones, and to act as shock absorbers in large weight-bearing joints such as the knee. Many synovial joints also have small sacs of fluid positioned in and around their different structures. These bursae cut down the friction between moving parts. There are six sub-types of synovial joints, with perhaps the best known being the ball-and-socket joints such as the shoulder and hip, and hinge joints such as the knee.

For movement to occur at joints, the joint in question must be structured in such a way that the required movement is possible in the first instance. For example, a hinge joint allows

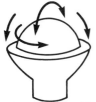
ball and socket e.g. hip joint

hinge e.g. knee joint

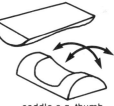
saddle e.g. thumb

ellipsoid e.g. wrist

pivot e.g. head/neck

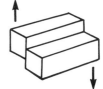
gliding e.g. wrist bones

Fig 2 Movements possible at the six sub-types of synovial joints.

11

movement in one plane only. Using the knee as an example, (although strictly speaking it is not a true hinge joint since some rotation is possible when the knee is flexed) you will see that it is possible to move the lower leg forwards and backwards only about the knee joint. At the hip joint (a ball-and-socket joint) it is possible to move the thigh forwards and backwards, and in all kinds of ways three-dimensionally. In other words, different joints are structured in such a way as to allow different movements. Trying to make a joint move through a range of movement for which it is not designed will inevitably lead to injury. Referring back to the knee joint again, imagine what would happen if the knee was forced sideways. This often happens in contact sports such as rugby football and can lead to massive joint damage as the knee is forced into a position it was not designed for. Less dramatically, it is also possible to weaken and damage a joint by persistently moving it into positions for which it was not designed, since even relatively slight movements out of the normal range of functioning of a joint can over-stretch the ligaments of a joint. If ligaments are over-stretched regularly they become abnormally lengthened and as a result, can no longer carry out their role of keeping bones together. The joint consequently becomes less stable, weaker, and more susceptible to injury. Such excessive joint laxity – in the wrong direction – at joints can quite easily be brought about through inappropriate stretching positions.

Accepting that a desired movement is possible at a joint, it is necessary for a muscle to begin above the joint and end below it if that movement is to occur. How a muscle produces force is very complex. Essentially however, muscle tissue is structured in such a way that when a muscle receives an appropriate nerve impulse, the muscle's fibres respond in such a way so that their ends are brought closer together. Muscle fibres are grouped together into bundles, with each bundle of muscle fibres being bound to the next with connective tissue. This connective tissue effectively runs around individual muscle fibres, bundles of muscle fibres and the muscle itself, finally coming together at the end of the muscle to form a strong cord of connective tissue which is known as a tendon, or a sheet of connective tissue which is known as an aponeurosis. The tendon or aponeurosis then attaches to bone or other connective tissues. It is through the tendon or aponeurosis that the muscle fibres exert their force upon bones, which being able to move at joints, end up producing the wide range of actions characteristic of the human body.

The above information hopefully indicates the importance of a sound knowledge of anatomy with respect to performing safe stretching movements. The following covers the major joints of the body and indicates the type of joint, the normal range of movement associated with each joint, and indicates the movements which are possible at each joint diagrammatically.

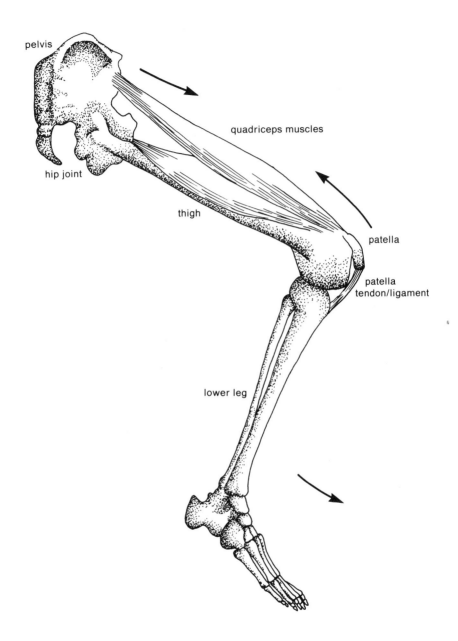

pelvis

quadriceps muscles

hip joint

thigh

patella

patella
tendon/ligament

lower leg

*Fig 3   How muscles produce movement. When the quadriceps muscle
contracts the ends are brought together; this causes extension at
the knee joint.*

Spinal Column *(Fig 4)*

Consists of a series of cartilaginous joints between successive vertebrae, plus two synovial joints and a synovial pivot joint at the top of the vertebral column which allows the head to flex, extend and rotate.

Viewed as a whole, the vertebral column allows the movements of:

i) flexion;
ii) extension;
iii) lateral flexion;
iv) rotation.

Flexion and extension are normally free in cervical (neck), thoracic (chest) and lumbar (lower back) regions. Lateral flexion is free in the cervical and lumbar regions but less free in the thoracic region. Rotation is most free at the top of the spine and least free at the bottom.

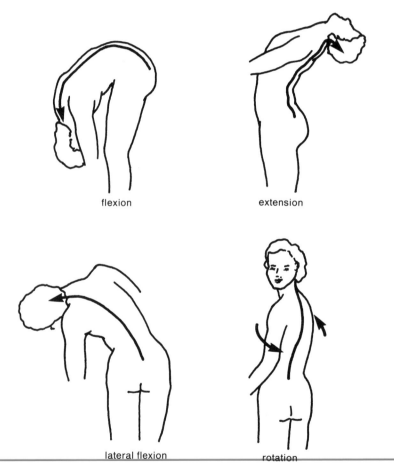

flexion

extension

lateral flexion

rotation

Fig 4   Movements of the spinal column.

Shoulder Girdle *(Fig 5)*

Each shoulder girdle consists of one scapula (shoulder blade) and one clavicle (collar bone). The basic movements of the shoulder girdles are:

i)   elevation;
ii)   depression;
iii) adduction (scapulae drawn towards the vertebral column);
iv)   abduction (scapulae drawn away from the vertebral column).

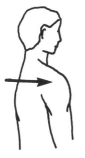

abduction

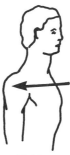

adduction

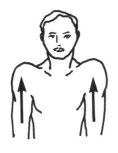

elevation

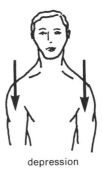

depression

Fig 5   Movements of the shoulder girdle.

15

Shoulder Joint *(Fig 6)*

The shoulder joint is a typical ball-and-socket joint; the 'ball' part is the end of the humerus. The movements which are possible at the shoulder joint are:

i) flexion;
ii) extension;
iii) adduction;
iv) abduction;
v) medial rotation;
vi) lateral rotation;
vii) circumduction.

Note that the degree of movement exhibited at the shoulder joint is much greater than that possible at the hip joint, which is also of a ball-and-socket type, since the socket at the shoulder joint is very shallow and the joint less powerfully constructed. The shoulder girdles can also move relatively freely around the rib-cage, unlike the more fixed pelvic girdle.

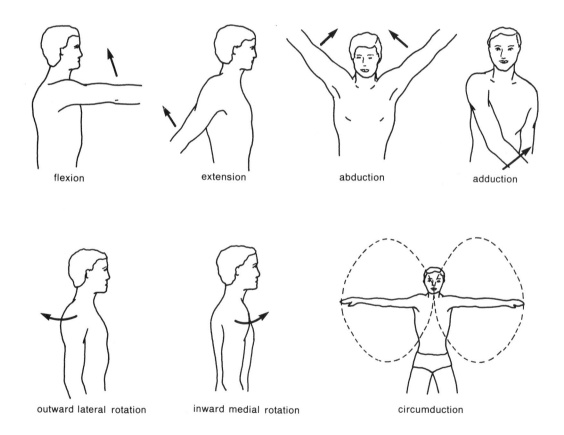

flexion extension abduction adduction

outward lateral rotation inward medial rotation circumduction

Fig 6 Movements of the shoulder joint.

Elbow Joint *(Fig 7)*

The elbow joint is classified as a hinge joint, although the bones of the forearm are arranged such that the forearm can rotate. The movements possible at the elbow joint are therefore:

i)   flexion;
ii) extension;
iii) pronation;
iv) supination.

Wrist Joint *(Fig 8)*

The wrist joint is a synovial joint (condyloid) which allows:

i)   flexion;
ii) extension;
iii) adduction;
iv) abduction;
v)   circumduction.

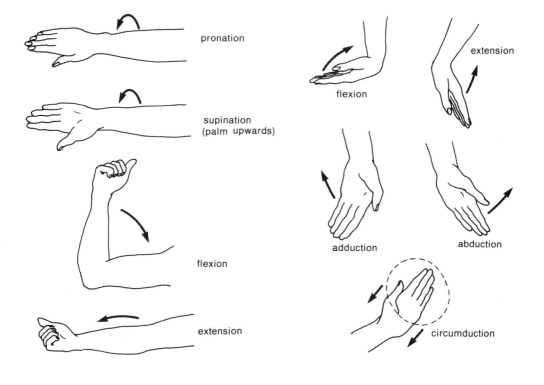

Fig 7   *Movements of the elbow joint.*

Fig 8   *Movements of the wrist joint.*

Hip Joint *(Fig 9)*

The hip joint is a ball-and-socket joint. It allows the following movements:

i)   flexion;
ii) extension;
iii) adduction;
iv) abduction;
v)   medial rotation;
vi) lateral rotation;
vii) circumduction.

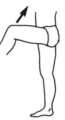
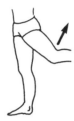

flexion   extension

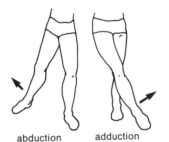

abduction   adduction

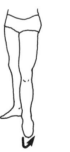
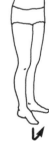

lateral rotation   medial rotation

Fig 9   Movements of the hip joint.

Knee Joint *(Fig 10)*

The knee joint is classified as a hinge joint, although as mentioned earlier, it permits some rotation when it is flexed. The movements at the knee joint are:

  i) flexion;
 ii) extension;
iii) medial rotation;
 iv) lateral rotation.

Ankle Joint *(Fig 11)*

The ankle joint is classified as a hinge joint and permits the movements of:

  i) plantar flexion ('true' extension);
 ii) dorsi flexion.

The joints between the various bones of the foot allow other movements, including:

iii) inversion;
 iv) eversion.

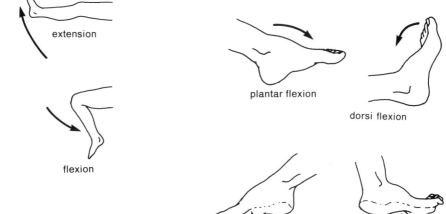

Fig 10   Movements of the knee joint.

Fig 11   Movements of the ankle and foot.

Using the above lists and diagrams, it should be clear just what movements should be possible at normal healthy joints in normal healthy individuals. Many of the above typical joint movements have in fact been used to enable exercise scientists to determine more exactly what the normal range of movement for an individual should be at each joint when compared to the average population. However, such exact measurements are time consuming and require a skilled technician and calibrated devices for measuring the angle through which a movement can be executed, such as a 'Leighton Flexometer'.

Simpler general assessments of your overall joint flexibility do exist, however, such as the following 'sit-and-reach test'. Such a test is only an indicator of general range of movement, though, since flexibility at a joint is specific to the joint in question, and what holds true for one joint in the body may not be the case for any other joint.

The Sit-and-Reach Test of General Flexibility *(Fig 12)*

This test is essentially an assessment of the flexibility of your lower back and hamstrings, although it is also considered to be a good indicator of general flexibility.

To perform the test you will need a box and a ruler. Fix the ruler to the top of the box with clear tape, so that half of the ruler projects over the edge of the box. Warm up thoroughly (*see* Chapter 4) and sit with your bare feet placed against the side of the box with your legs straight, as illustrated in *Fig 12*. Reach as far forward as possible with outstretched fingers (do not bounce) and note how far along the ruler your fingertips are. Distances past the edge of the box should be recorded as 'plus' values, whilst distances in front of the edge of the box should be recorded as 'minus' values. Compare your score on the best of three attempts using the scoring table (*Fig 13*).

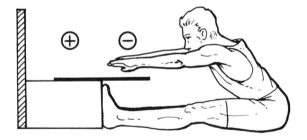

Fig 12   The sit-and-reach test of general flexibility.

SCORING TABLE FOR THE SIT-AND-REACH TEST	
Excellent	+ 15cm
Good	+ 10cm
Fair	+ 5cm
Average	0cm
Poor	less than 0cm

Fig 13

As useful as this test is for assessing your general flexibility, such an assessment does not say much about how limited your movement may be at other joints. To circumvent this problem, a simple series of muscle tightness tests have been designed by Drs Peter and Lorna Francis at San Diego State University. The seven simple tests look at the range of movement in the shoulders, lower back, front of the hips, back of the thighs, front of the thighs and calves and require you to aim for a specific goal. If you meet that goal, you can assume that your overall range of movement is more than adequate. If not, then a specific stretching programme is needed! These tests, along with the sit-and-reach test should tell you all you need to know about your flexibility and range of movement. Repeat them, say every few weeks, to gauge the effectiveness of your stretching programme.

The Muscle Tightness Tests *(Figs 14–16)*

In each case, ease into the stretch position as far as possible, registering mild discomfort, perhaps, but never pain. Never force or bounce a limb into any of the positions illustrated.

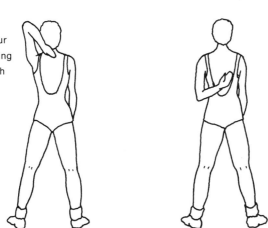

try to touch the top of your shoulder blade by reaching backwards and down with one arm to the opposite shoulder blade

try to touch the bottom of your shoulder blade by reaching backwards and up with one arm to the opposite shoulder blade

Figs 14–16   The flexibility tests devised by Drs Peter and Lorna Francis.

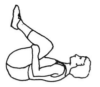

try to pull your knees to your chest
while lying on your back

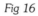

lie on your stomach with your knees
together and pull one heel towards
your buttocks – it should be
comfortably done

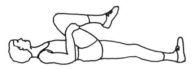

lie on your back with one leg extended and bring the
other leg to your chest; the calf of your extended leg
must remain on the floor and the knee of this leg
must not bend

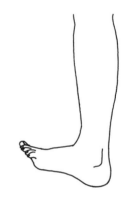

stand with your heels, buttocks and back against
a wall and raise one forefoot off the floor by the
width at least of two fingers; keep both knees
straight but relaxed and your heels down

Fig 16

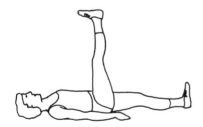

lie on your back and raise one leg to a vertical
position, keeping the other flat on the floor;
do not bend either knee

Fig 15

3 Methods of Stretching

There are currently several different methods of stretching commonly used by athletes and sportspeople to increase their range of movement. These various techniques of stretching may be grouped under the following headings:

ballistic methods;
static methods;
assisted methods.

BALLISTIC METHODS OF STRETCHING

Essentially, for any exercise to be classified as a 'stretch' all that exercise needs to do is to take a limb and its associated muscles and joints into a position it has not been in before. Ballistic methods of stretching achieve this through fairly vigorous and sometimes forced actions. For example, a ballistic technique designed to stretch the hamstrings would involve positioning yourself as for the sit-and-reach flexibility test (see Chapter 2). Once in this position, you would then try and 'bounce' further forward towards your toes a number of times in succession.

Ballistic methods of stretching, involving some form of rapid movement into a stretch position have been popular for many years. Indeed, some of the earliest systematic physical training employed in schools and colleges involved ballistic exercise methods. Ballistic stretching, however, has fallen from favour lately – forced, rapid stretching techniques do seem to be associated with increased damage and soreness to muscles and connective tissues in general. The reason for this high incidence

of injury when performing ballistic exercise – and how to avoid injury when exercising ballistically – is explained in the second part of this chapter.

Despite the bad press that ballistic stretching has received in the last few years it is well worth pointing out that ballistic methods for improving ranges of movement do work. It is also worth further mention that ballistic movements are an essential aspect of many sports techniques. Because of this, practising some ballistic movements at the right time in your conditioning session may well be necessary if you are to avoid subsequent injury during competition or sports performance.

STATIC METHODS OF STRETCHING

Unlike ballistic methods of stretching, static methods of stretching, as the name implies, involve little movement as such. Instead, stretch positions are eased into and held. For example, stretching the hamstrings using the sit-and-reach flexibility test position in *Fig12*, would mean that having reached as far forward towards your toes as possible, you would then hold that furthermost position for a given period of time. The amount of time the static position is held varies, but may be anything between six seconds and two minutes. Often in static stretching you are advised to move further into the position of stretch as the sensation of stretch subsides.

Static methods of stretching produce excellent results. Static stretching has been shown to improve flexibility more than ballistic stretching, generally speaking, although some researchers have found both methods equally effective in increasing ranges of movement. However, all researchers are agreed that static methods of stretching produce far fewer instances of muscle soreness, injury and damage to connective tissues than ballistic methods.

ASSISTED METHODS OF STRETCHING

Assisted methods of stretching are becoming more and more widespread. In most assisted methods you require the help of a partner (although gravity and various new exercise devices may be employed which effectively take the place of a partner). Taking the hamstrings as an example of a muscle group to be stretched again, and using a partner, you would assume the position as illustrated: back flat, shoulders and upper body relaxed, leg flexed at the hip to approximately ninety degrees, knee extended and ankle dorsi flexed. Your partner positions himself or herself so that he or she can push against the back of your leg.

From this position there are a variety of techniques which can be performed, all of which have been called proprioceptive neuromuscular facilitation (PNF) techniques. One of the most common PNF techniques is referred to as slow-reversal hold. Referring to the above position, your partner eases your leg forward to a position when you can feel a slight discomfort – this is not pain! When this point is reached, you then push against your partner by strongly contracting the hamstring muscles which have just been stretched. Your partner does not allow your leg to move. After a count of ten, you then relax your hamstring muscles, contract your quadricep muscles (those on the front of the thigh) and your partner applies pressure to your leg again to ease it, if possible, further forward into the stretch position. After ten seconds of partner pressure, the sequence is repeated again, usually at least three times.

Other PNF techniques are just variations on this theme. Such assisted methods have been shown to produce quite dramatic increases in ranges of movement, improvements which are often considerably greater than those achieved through either ballistic or static methods. However, the real risk of injury is again present, since a partner who is not sympathetic to your needs can cause you to injure yourself. For this reason assisted stretching should not be undertaken lightly, or over-enthusiastically. It needs to be careful and considered, with both partners fully understanding the technique and the rationale behind it.

THE PHYSIOLOGY UNDERLYING THE VARIOUS STRETCHING METHODS

The reasons for the potential injury associated with ballistic methods of stretching, and the apparent effectiveness of static and PNF techniques are relatively easily understood when the role of various receptors in the muscles and tendons and neurophysiological phenomena in general are explained.

Firstly, all muscles contain receptors which are known as muscle spindles. The role of a particular muscle spindle is to pick up information about the length and rate of change of length of the muscle in which that spindle is found. So, for example, when a muscle is being lengthened (stretched) the information about the change in length of the muscle is picked up by the muscle spindle and relayed to the central nervous system (in this case the spinal cord). The automatic reflex response is to send a nerve impulse to the muscle which is changing length, telling it to contract. This sequence of events may in this instance be considered as a safety mechanism, aimed at preventing the muscle which is undergoing the rapid stretch from stretching too far and being subsequently damaged. It is worth noting that the speed at which the muscle is lengthened is crucial: the more rapidly the muscle changes length, the more forceful the reflex response causing the same muscle to contract.

Tendons of muscles also contain specialised receptors which are referred to as Golgi tendon organs (GTOs). The role of the GTO is to register information about the degree of tension in the tendon and hence in the muscle associated with that tendon. The reflex response which occurs as a result of stimulation of the GTO is to cause the muscle in which high tension is being registered to relax. Again, this may be considered to be something of a safety valve, since when the muscle relaxes, the high tension within that muscle and its tendon (which could damage the muscle and/or its connective tissues) will decrease.

Also of interest is the fact that when a muscle contracts, its opposing muscle group (that which produces the opposite action or movement) relaxes – this process is known as reciprocal innervation.

In the light of this information, the injury problems associated with ballistic stretching can clearly be appreciated. The very rapid changes in length brought about through forced, bounced movements stimulate the muscle's spindles. In turn, a reflex contraction (or shortening) of the muscle being lengthened occurs. Effectively, such forced, bounced movements cause the body to fight against itself, as it attempts to resist rapid changes in limb position through muscular contractions. However, once a limb is accelerated, simple physics indicates that massive forces are necessary to halt its movement. The potential for damaging muscles and tendons then becomes apparent.

The effectiveness of static stretching methods, and the almost complete lack of injury associated with such techniques (when correctly executed) is largely a result of stimulation of the GTOs. As a static stretch position is held, the tension registered by the GTO in a stretched muscle tendon leads to a reflex relaxation of the muscle being stretched. This means that it then becomes possible to ease further forward into the stretch position – a phenomenon which can be observed by anyone who maintains a stretch position for any length of time. It would appear that the stretch position has to be held for upwards of six seconds, preferably longer, for the inhibitory signals from the GTOs to override excitatory impulses from the muscle spindles before relaxation occurs.

Obviously, PNF techniques take advantage of these mechanisms and that of reciprocal innervation. The sustained stretch of the muscle first leads to relaxation as in a static stretch. The next phase of muscular contraction then increases the tension in the muscle/tendon, (since tension will be generated in the muscle/tendon both when a muscle is being lengthened and when it is contracting) so that further GTO stimulation occurs. This leads to further relaxation when the contraction phase ends and the limb is eased into the stretch position by the partner. The strong contraction of the opposing muscle group also leads to reciprocal innervation and potential for the muscle group being stretched to lengthen still further.

WHICH METHOD IS BEST?

For general, all-round effectiveness and for ease of performance, static stretching is probably the best stretching method for most people. Static stretching carries a very low injury risk, is relatively simple to carry out and does not require the help of a partner – and static stretches may be performed virtually anywhere. Many sportsmen and women find, for example, that it is easy enough to slot in a considerable amount of stretching whilst watching the television.

For maximum gains in flexibility in the shortest possible time, however, a PNF technique may be the preferred choice, as long as the method employed as discussed earlier, is performed intelligently and with the help of a knowledgeable, experienced partner. Readers who are keen to try a modified PNF technique should refer to the guide-lines given in Chapter 5.

Finally, ballistic stretching may be necessary in some instances. Take the example of performing any rapid sports movement, like kicking a football. It was pointed out in Chapter 1 that achieving any great distance with a football kick requires force to be applied at the right angle throughout the greatest possible distance or range of movement. It is also necessary to accelerate the kicking foot as much as possible throughout that range of movement. In essence, any rapid action such as this is a ballistic one, and many muscles will be lengthened very rapidly. To avoid injury in the performance of such a ballistic technique, it is vital that the body is prepared for the ballistic action which is to follow. This can be achieved by warming the body up thoroughly, then carrying out appropriate preparatory static stretches. This sequence of stretching should then be followed by a progressive series of ballistic movements, similar to the sports activity itself. Start off with the movement or activity at half speed for a few repetitions, then increase the speed gradually, working up to an all-out performance of the activity itself. Such progressive and specific preparation will ensure that the risk of injury to muscles, joints and joint structures is minimised.

Obviously, it is quite possible to combine all the techniques and methods of stretching outlined if desired. If there are occasions when you are fortunate enough to be able to work with a partner, then PNF stretching could be the order of the day, taking the place of your normal static stretching programme. However, to reiterate, for most people static stretching is probably the safest, most effective option for an increase in overall range of movement.

4 Designing a Stretching Programme

Designing an exercise programme to improve an individual's range of movement follows the same rules and guide-lines in general that any exercise or training programme must do if it is to achieve its end result safely.

Essentially, the programme of exercise must overload the body with an appropriate stimulus both long enough and often enough. Provided these rules are followed and bearing in mind the information presented in the previous chapters, a marked increase in an individual's range of movement will be seen in just a few short weeks.

The appropriate stimulus for an increase in the range of movement at a joint is that of taking a limb and its associated muscles, joints and joint structures into a position it has not been in before. This position, as has been indicated, must be anatomically sound, and if possible, should be maintained for at least six seconds if the muscle being stretched is to relax more fully, in accordance with what has been said about the role of muscle spindles and GTOs. It would appear that six seconds is about the minimum that a static position should be held for an increase in range of movement to take place. Some authorities have advocated holding a static position for longer than this, even up to two minutes, yet for increasing flexibility, thirty seconds of developmental stretching is probably more than adequate. Without measuring devices, the only effective way of knowing whether you are in a position which you have not been in before is to rely upon what your body is telling you.

The 'sensation of stretch' which has been referred to in the text is one of very mild discomfort in the particular muscle group being stretched. It is not one of pain, nor is it sharp or stabbing in nature. As the stretch position is held, you should also notice that the sensation of discomfort subsides. When it does, ease further forward into the stretch exercise position until you feel exactly the same level of slight discomfort. This is the sensation of stretch you should be looking for when you carry out each exercise. As an aid, you will note that the instructions accompanying the stretching exercises later on in the book state exactly where you should feel the stretch. Use this information, along with the rest of the instructions, to ensure that you are carrying the exercise out correctly.

The length of time each stretch should be held for depends largely upon why you are stretching and your current level of fitness. For example, during static stretching as part of the warm-up phase prior to exercise, the preparatory stretches need only be held for approximately six seconds. Here the aim is not to develop flexibility as such, but to take the body through its current range of movement, in preparation for more strenuous physical activity. However, when it comes to increasing flexibility longer stretches must be employed – these are the thirty second duration, developmental stretches.

Initially, only one developmental stretch for each major muscle group may be necessary. Yet as your body adapts, you will find that you will have to either hold the stretches for longer, if you are keen on further improvement, or that you need to repeat the stretches in sequence, rather like you would repeat a sequence of weight-training exercises. Three circuits of thirty-second developmental stretches for all major muscle groups in the body is an excellent regime for overall increases in flexibility.

Note that stretching is joint specific. In other words, you will only see improvements in the range of movement of the joint you exercise. General increases in flexibility require a variety of different stretching exercises for all the major muscle groups. However, you can, if your needs dictate, structure a stretching programme targeting specific problem areas. Examples of general and specific stretching programmes are given in Chapter 7.

It is also necessary to ensure that the body has been sufficiently warmed and 'loosened up' prior to stretching. Not only does this ensure that the stretches will be carried out with little injury risk, but it is also well documented that muscles and joints are more responsive to a stretching programme when they are warm. Because of this, this chapter also contains detailed information on how to warm up prior to engaging in a stretching programme. Obviously, if you have been exercising vigorously your body will already be very warm and ready for a stretching programme. Research has shown that after a session of relatively vigorous physical activity and provided the body is not subject to rapid cooling, then it is possible to stretch safely for as much as forty-five minutes following the end of your activity phase. However, it probably makes sense to cool down for a few minutes only, then start your stretching programme, since, as pointed out in Chapter 1, the anecdotal evidence supports the role of stretching exercises following strenuous training in the prevention of muscle stiffness and soreness.

Finally, what kind of changes in flexibility should you expect? Obviously this depends upon all kinds of factors, not least of which is you as an individual. The ultimate limiting factor in mobility is the structure of your joints – this differs from person to person. However, it does

seem possible for appropriate stretching programmes to lead to increases in joint movement of several degrees brought about mainly through considerable elongation of the fascial sheath surrounding the muscles. Yet it should also be remembered that old injuries may mean that your range of movement at a specific joint may always be limited more than normal.

However, improvement will only be seen if you take your starting position into account. Perform the assessment exercises in Chapter 2 before beginning your stretching programme and compare how you score on each test every four weeks.

WARMING UP

It has already been stated that the body responds best to a stretching programme when it is warm. Indeed, the body responds best to any exercise activity following a warm-up phase. This is because increasing the temperature of the body leads to a number of favourable physiological responses as far as movement and exercises are concerned. Muscles, for example, find it easier to contract and relax, since their viscosity (or 'stickiness') is reduced as their temperature increases. Nerve impulses can also travel more readily and be received more quickly, the response of the heart to exercise is improved, oxygen is made more available to the muscles for energy release and overall, the likelihood of damage to muscles, tendons and joints is greatly reduced when the body is warm.

There are basically two methods of warming up, namely passive and active. Passive methods of warming up rely upon some form of heat source – this may be a heat lamp, warm bath or shower, radiator, sauna and the like. Active methods of warming up rely upon the fact that when muscles perform work (that is contract or cause movement) they generate a large amount of heat. Also, during exercise, large amounts of blood are moved to working muscles. This extra blood flow further leads to an increase in muscle temperature, since blood can act like an internal central heating system, carrying heat around the body.

Whilst both methods of warming up will lead to an increase in temperature, it is generally agreed that in most cases, active methods are preferable since deep muscle temperature seems to be increased more readily than with passive methods. Active methods can also be made more relevant to the exercise and physical activity which is to follow the warm-up phase. However, there is no reason why you should not combine active and passive methods to achieve the most appropriate warm-up for you and your situation.

Whichever method or methods you choose, your warm-up phase prior to stretching should have two aims: to increase the temperature of the body; and to take muscles and joints through their current range of movement. Effectively, at the end of your warm-up phase, your body should feel 'ready for action'. Generally, the onset of light sweating and a feeling of looseness are good indicators of a thorough warm-up. These effects can be achieved by most people in five to ten minutes, although older or more unfit people may find that they have to exercise for longer to achieve the full benefits of warming up. Athletes and sportsmen whose activity is very explosive may also find that a longer warm-up period is necessary for them to perform at their best. It is also worth bearing in mind that the ambient temperature can also determine how your warm-up phase is structured. In very warm weather, the amount of time spent increasing the temperature of the body can be decreased, and the emphasis instead placed upon taking muscles and joints throughout their

full ranges of movement. The opposite is, of course, the case if it is particularly cold. Loose layers of clothing can also be used to great advantage when warming up, since layers of T-shirts, track suits and the like can trap the heat that the body is producing, enabling an increase in general temperature to occur more readily.

The following warming-up sequence should suit the purposes of most people. The sequence assumes that there are no special facilities available and prepares the exerciser for a general developmental stretching programme. Alternatively, the sequence can be used as a warm-up prior to a general fitness or training session.

GENERAL WARM-UP SEQUENCE

Dress in warm, loose layers of clothing (according to the enviromental temperature) which allow full freedom of movement. Wear suitable footwear and perform all exercises in a well-ventilated space.

Start your warm-up sequence by checking your posture. Your feet should be a comfortable distance apart (approximately shoulder width) and your weight should be evenly balanced. Your pelvis should feel 'centred' (buttocks tucked under slightly) and your spine long. Aim to have your shoulders down away from your ears, with your arms loosely by your sides. Feel tall, yet relaxed. (More information on posture is included in Chapter 6.)

Bearing the above postural pointers in mind, now perform the following sequence of mobilising exercises. Read each instruction carefully before you perform the exercise and do not bounce, jerk or force yourself into any position.

Shoulder Circles *(Fig 17)*

Stand tall with good posture. Raise your right shoulder towards your right ear, take it backwards, down and then up again with a smooth rhythm. Perform this shoulder circling movement eight times, then repeat with the other shoulder. Breathe easily throughout the sequence.

Arm Circles *(Fig 18)*

Stand tall with good posture. Lift one arm forward then take it backwards in a continuous circling motion, keeping your spine long throughout. Perform this arm circling movement eight times, before repeating with the other arm. Avoid the tendency to arch your spine whilst carrying out the circling movement. Breathe easily throughout.

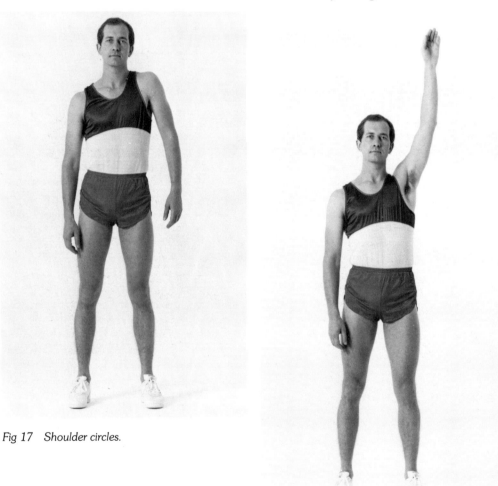

Fig 17   Shoulder circles.

Fig 18   Arm circles.

Side Bends *(Fig 19)*

Stand tall with good posture, feet slightly wider than shoulder-width apart, knees slightly bent, hands resting on hips. Lift your trunk up and away from your hips and bend smoothly first to one side, then the other, avoiding the tendency to lean either forwards or backwards. Repeat the whole sequence sixteen times with a slow rhythm, breathing out as you bend to the side, and in as you return to the centre.

Trunk Twists *(Fig 20)*

Stand tall with good posture. Have your feet slightly wider than hip-width apart, knees slightly bent, hands resting on hips. Keeping your spine long and your hips facing forward, turn smoothly and slowly round to one side, then the other. Repeat the sequence sixteen times, breathing easily throughout the movement.

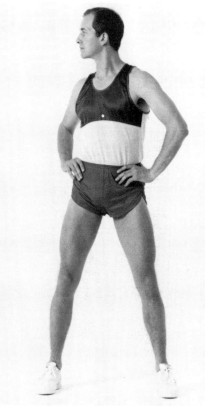

Fig 20   Trunk twists.

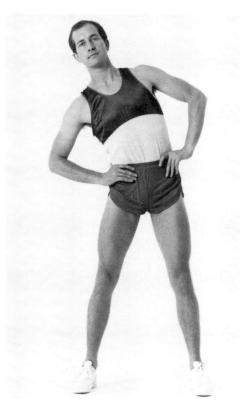

Fig 19   Side bends.

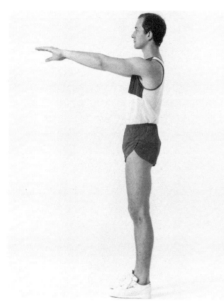

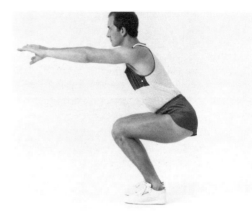

Fig 22

Figs 21 & 22   Half squat

Half Squat *(Figs 21 and 22)*

Stand tall with good posture, holding your hands out in front of you for balance. Now bend at the knees until your thighs are parallel with the floor. Keep your back long throughout the movement, and look straight ahead. Make sure that your knees always point in the same direction as your toes. Once at your lowest point, fully straighten your legs to return to your starting position. Repeat the exercise sixteen times with a smooth, controlled rhythm. Breathe in as you descend, and out as you rise.

The above exercises should leave you feeling reasonably warm and relatively loose. If you have the option, light jogging, cycling, rowing or any other exercise activity performed at low intensity for five minutes will further ensure that you are warmed-up sufficiently to exercise safely. The next stage is to perform the preparatory stretches listed in the general stretching programme on page 88. Read the instructions for each stretch carefully, and hold each stretch

position for just six seconds, before moving on to the next stretch. Having performed all the preparatory stretches, you are then ready to begin your developmental stretching in earnest, or to begin your work-out or training session. If the latter is the case, at the end of your training phase, ease down with light rhythmical movements, keep warm (replace track suits and the like if necessary) and then continue with your developmental stretching, as before.

THE STRETCHES

This section of the book contains all the stretches which are needed in order to perform any of the stretching programmes listed throughout the text. The stretches here are static ones and may be used as either preparatory or developmental exercises according to the length of time for which they are held. For preparatory stretching, ease into your furthermost stretch position and hold it for six seconds. For developmental stretching, ease into the stretch position and hold it for thirty seconds, moving further into the exercise position as the sensation of stretch subsides. For further information on PNF stretching exercises, *see* Chapter 5.

Note: Read all the instructions carefully before attempting any of the exercises.

Whilst performing all exercises, bear in mind your posture and the position that all of your joints are in – are your limbs moving through the appropriate ranges of movement as described in Chapter 2?

STRETCHES FOR THE LOWER LEG

The basic movements possible at the ankle joint are plantar and dorsi flexion. The main muscles involved in these movements are the gastrocnemius and soleus (plantar flexion) and tibialis anterior (dorsi flexion).

Standing Calf Stretch (Gastrocnemius) *(Fig 23)*

Stand tall with one leg in front of the other, hands flat and at shoulder height against a wall or suitable immovable object. Ease your back

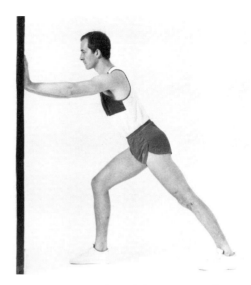

Fig 23   Standing calf stretch (gastrocnemius).

leg further away from the wall, keeping it straight and press the heel firmly into the floor. Keep your hips facing the wall. You will feel the stretch in the calf of the rear leg (*see Fig 24*). Repeat on the other side. Breathe easily throughout the exercise.

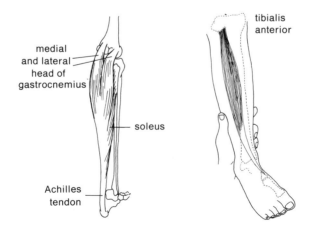

medial and lateral head of gastrocnemius

soleus

Achilles tendon

tibialis anterior

Fig 24   Muscles of the lower leg.

Standing Calf Stretch (Soleus) *(Fig 25)*

Position yourself as for the previous exercise. This time, however, flex the knee of the rear leg, whilst still keeping the heel pressed firmly on to the floor. The sensation of stretch should now be experienced lower down in the calf. Repeat on the other side, breathing easily throughout.

Free-standing Calf Stretch (Gastrocnemius and Soleus) *(Fig 26)*

In the absence of a wall or object to lean against, you can stretch the calf muscles by standing with one foot in front of the other as illustrated, making sure that you have a firm, stable base of support, with feet facing forwards. From this position, bend both knees, whilst keeping your spine long and looking straight ahead. You will feel the stretch in the calf of the back leg. Repeat with the other leg, breathing easily throughout.

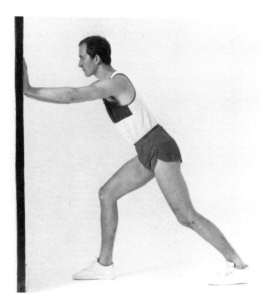

Fig 25   *Standing calf stretch (soleus).*

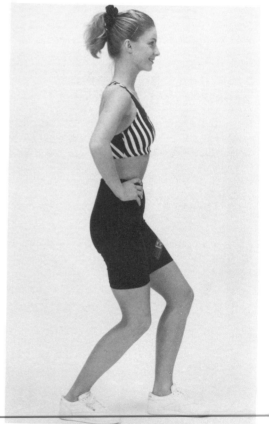

Fig 26   *Free-standing calf stretch.*

34

Kerb Stretch (Gastrocnemius) *(Fig 27)*

You can also stretch the calf very effectively using a kerb or step. Stand with the ball of your foot on the edge of the step and ease your heels towards the floor, feeling the stretch in the calf and breathing easily throughout the exercise. You can perform this movement with both legs at the same time, or with individual legs.

Front of Lower Leg Stretch (Tibialis Anterior) *(Fig 28)*

To stretch the front of the lower leg and foot sit upright in a chair with one of your legs underneath the chair as illustrated – this exercise is best performed without shoes. With your toes pointed, press your foot down and forward against the floor, feeling the stretch along the front of the lower leg and foot. Repeat the movement with the other leg, breathing easily throughout.

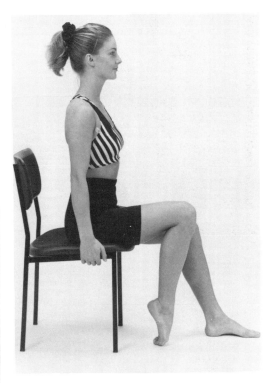

Fig 28   Front of lower leg stretch.

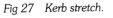

Fig 27   Kerb stretch.

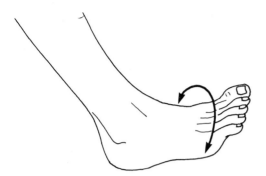

Having performed any or all of the above stretches, you may like to circle your feet in both directions several times *(Fig 29)*, and invert and evert your feet several times *(Fig 30)* as well as flexing and extending your toes *(Fig 31)*. Try also to spread your toes as far apart as possible, so that there is a space between adjoining toes *(Fig 32)*. Simple movements like these will help to keep your feet flexible.

Fig 29   Foot circling.

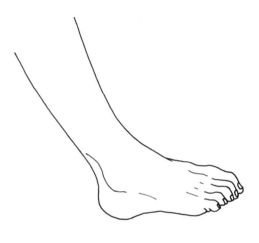

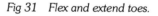

Fig 31   Flex and extend toes.

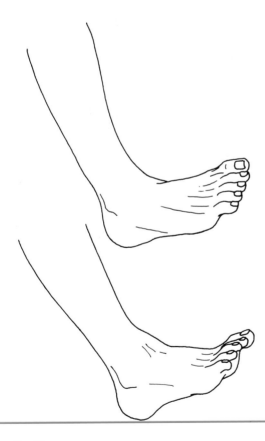

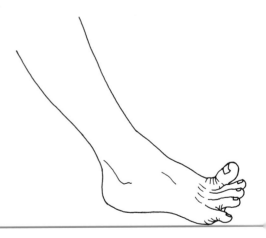

Fig 30   Invert and evert feet.

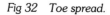

Fig 32   Toe spread.

STRETCHES FOR THE UPPER LEG

The basic movements possible at the knee joint are flexion and extension, although some rotation is possible when the knee is flexed. The muscles which produce extension at the knee joint are the quadriceps group (vastus medialis, vastus intermedius, vastus lateralis and rectus femoris). The muscles which produce flexion at this joint are the hamstring group (biceps femoris, semitendinous, semimembranosus).

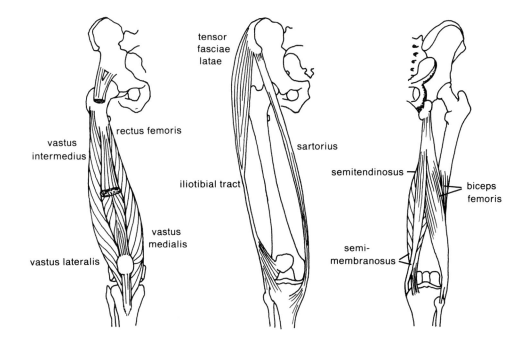

Fig 33 *Muscles of the thigh.*

Standing Quadriceps Stretch *(Fig 34)*

Stand tall with good posture. Hold on to the back of a chair for support and reach behind yourself with your right arm to loosely grasp your right foot. Gently ease your foot towards your buttocks, keeping your spine long and your pelvis tucked under, hips facing forward. Aim to have your knees alongside each other. You will feel the stretch along the front of the thigh. Repeat on the other side, breathing easily throughout. If you have difficulty performing this movement initially, try beginning the exercise with the knee of the supporting leg flexed slightly. Gradually try and straighten your support leg as the stretch progresses.

Note: It is very important in this exercise that you do not overarch the lumbar spine. The exercise is much more effective if you keep your pelvis tucked under.

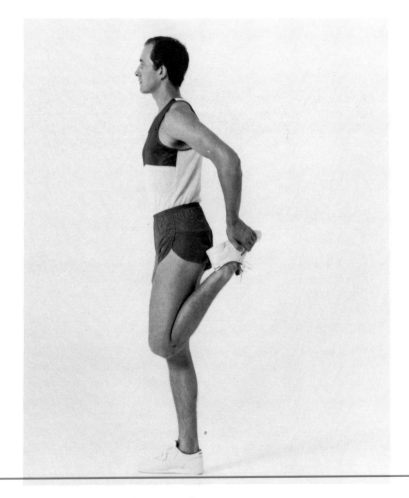

Fig 34 Standing quadriceps stretch.

Lying Quadriceps Stretch *(Fig 35)*

Lie face down on the floor, resting your forehead on your right hand. Press your hips firmly into the floor and bring your left foot up towards your buttocks, easing it closer to them with your right hand. You will feel the stretch along the front of the thigh. Repeat on the other side, breathing easily throughout the exercise.

There are many variations of these front-of-thigh stretches – these are by far the simplest and safest for the quadriceps group.

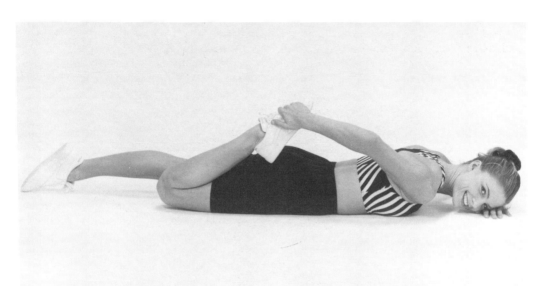

Fig 35   Lying quadriceps stretch.

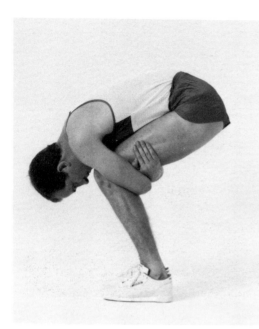

Figs 36 & 37 Standing hamstring stretch.

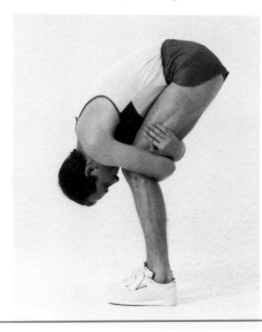

Standing Hamstring Stretch *(Figs 36 and 37)*

Stand tall with good posture. Now flex at the knees and hips until you can easily rest your chest on your thighs. Reach round with your arms and grasp your calves to bring your chest and thighs firmly together. From this position, try and straighten your legs as much as possible, whilst still keeping your chest firmly pressed against your thighs. When you reach your furthermost position you will feel the stretch along the backs of your thighs. Release the stretch by flexing the knees. Breathe easily throughout the movement.

Lying Hamstring Stretch *(Fig 38)*

Lie flat on the floor with your knees flexed to approximately ninety degrees. Raise your left leg, grasping it loosely behind the thigh with both hands. Now ease this leg as close to your chest as possible, keeping your other leg straight along the floor. You will feel the stretch along the back of the flexed thigh. Repeat with the other leg. Breathe easily throughout. If you can perform this exercise relatively easily, then go back to your original starting position and this time try and straighten your raised leg, before easing it closer towards your chest *(Fig 39)*. Again, you will feel the stretch along the back of the raised thigh, although this time you will experience the sensation of stretch throughout the length of the thigh, and not just towards the top, as in the previous exercise. In both exercises, keep your back flat along the length of the floor. Repeat with the other leg. Breathe easily throughout the movement.

Fig 37

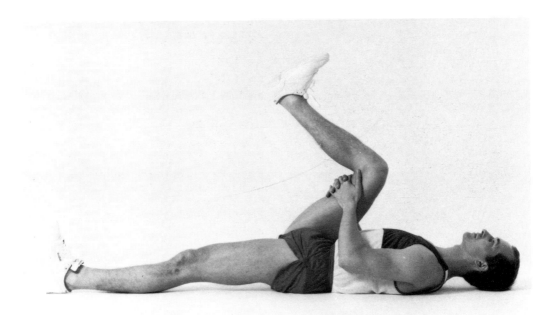

Fig 38   Lying hamstring stretch.

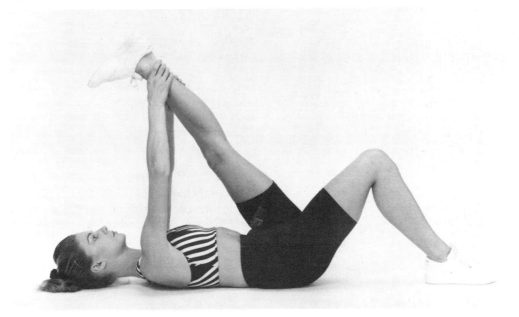

Fig 39   Lying hamstring stretch variation.

There are several variations of the above positions. The easier lying hamstring stretch can be varied by changing the position of the lower leg as illustrated in *Fig 40*. Do not pull forcefully on the lower leg, however, but ease it into position. You will feel the stretch further round to the outside of the back of the thigh.

Similarly, if you can perform the exercise shown in *Fig 39* with relative ease, you can combine the exercise with a movement for the inner thigh muscles as illustrated (*Fig 41*).

Several exercises for the hamstring muscles also involve the lower back. For example the sit-and-reach test of general flexibility is basically an assessment of hamstring and lower back mobility. It can also be used as an exercise in its own right, by reaching forward with outstretched legs and relaxed spine to loosely grasp your lower legs, ankles or feet according to your range of movement (*Fig 42*).

Other combined hamstring and other muscle group stretches include the following:

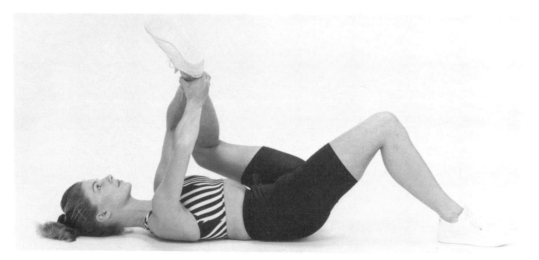

Fig 40   *Lying hamstring stretch variation.*

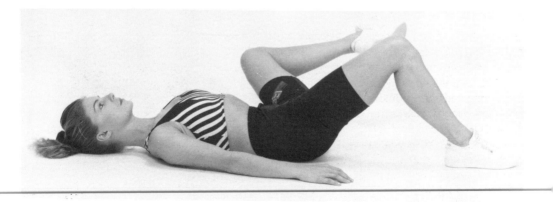

Fig 41   *Lying hamstring stretch variation.*

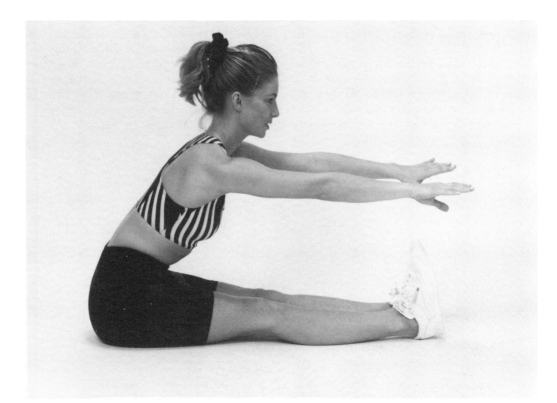

Fig 42   Seated hamstring/lower back stretch.

Seated Hamstring and Groin Stretch *(Fig 43)*

Sit tall with both legs fully outstretched. Flex your right knee so that the right foot rests comfortably along your left inner thigh, with the right knee as close as possible to the floor. Keeping your spine long and your shoulders down away from your ears, hinge forwards from the hips to reach towards your flexed left foot. Go as far forward as possible, then relax your spine to reach even further forward, holding this stretch position. You will feel the stretch along the back of the outstretched leg, and along the inside and rear of the flexed leg. Repeat with the other leg, breathing easily throughout.

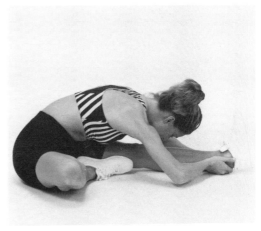

Fig 43   Seated hamstring and groin stretch.

Standing Hip and Thigh Stretch *(Fig 44)*

This exercise also stretches the muscles of the front of the thigh, specifically the rectus femoris. Stand tall with good posture in front of a firm chair or stool. Raise one foot up on to the chair back easing your body towards this foot so that chest and thigh come closer together. Rest your hands loosely on the raised knee and keep your spine and back leg straight and your shoulders down away from your ears. Ease as far forward as possible and hold your position. You will feel the stretch along the front of the thigh of the extended leg, and along the back of the thigh of the raised leg. Repeat on the other side, breathing easily throughout.

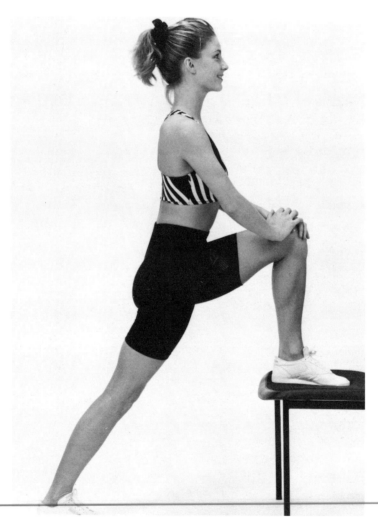

Fig 44   Standing hip and thigh stretch.

STRETCHES FOR THE MUSCLES OF THE HIP JOINT

There are six basic movements which are possible at the hip joint. These are flexion, extension, adduction, abduction, medial rotation and lateral rotation. A seventh movement – circumduction – which is a combination of the six basic movements is also possible. Note that in many instances, joint actions will be combined, for example as in crossing the legs. This action is a combination of flexion, abduction and lateral rotation as far as the hip joint is concerned. *Fig 48* summarises which muscles produce which action. For ease of description, muscles which produce hip extension will subsequently be referred to as 'hip extensors', those which produce flexion, as 'hip flexors' and so on.

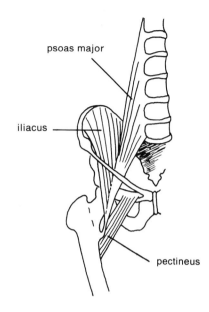

Fig 45   The deep hip flexor muscles.

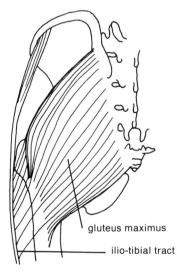

Fig 46   The gluteal muscles.

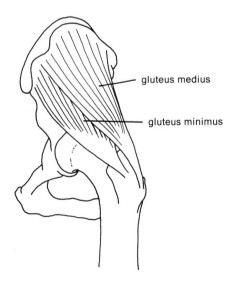

45

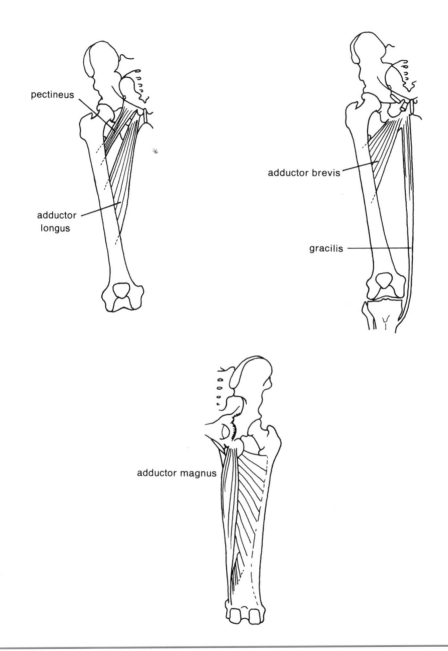

Fig 47   *The adductor muscles of the thigh.*

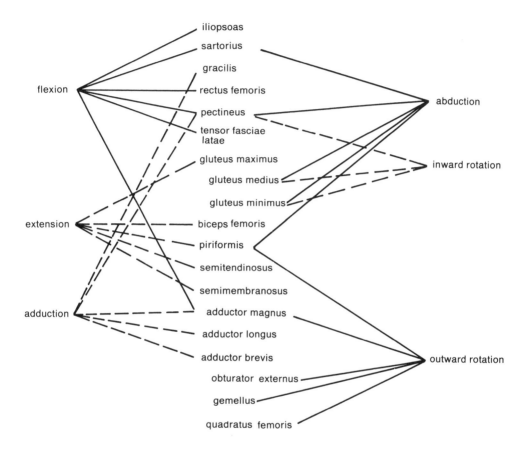

Fig 48   Movements at the hip joint and the muscles which produce those movements.

Kneeling Hip Flexor Stretch *(Fig 49)*

Kneel on a mat or towel with one leg flexed in front of you as illustrated – your weight should be evenly distributed so that your position is stable, although you can use your hands at either side of your body for extra support. Note that the knee of the front leg is positioned directly over the front foot. From this position and keeping your spine long and shoulders down, push your hips forward. You may find that you have to take your rear knee further back before you can feel the stretch along the front of this thigh. Repeat on the other side, breathing easily throughout the exercise.

Lying Hip Flexor Stretch *(Fig 50)*

This exercise requires a plank of wood and small blocks of wood of varying thicknesses. Place the plank on the floor and raise one end of it using a wood block so that it is elevated by approximately one inch. Lie with your back on the plank so that your hips are just at the edge of the raised end and keep your lower back and shoulders pressed firmly against the plank. Keep your legs straight and have your heels resting on the floor. You will feel the stretch along the front of both

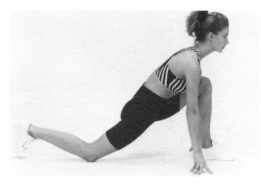

Fig 49   Kneeling hip flexor stretch.

thighs. Breathe easily throughout the exercise. As your flexibility improves you can raise the end of the plank further. However, never elevate the end of the plank so much that you cannot keep your lower back pressed firmly against the support.

Another useful hip flexor stretch is the standing hip and thigh stretch as shown in *Fig 44*.

Many stretches for the hamstring muscles are also stretches for the hip extensors in general, since the hamstring muscles aid the gluteus maximus in producing this movement. These exercises include the standing hamstring stretch *(Figs 36 and 37)*, the seated hamstring and groin stretch *(Fig 43)* and the standing hip and thigh stretch *(Fig 44)*.

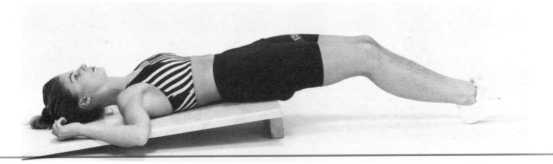

Fig 50   Lying hip flexor stretch.

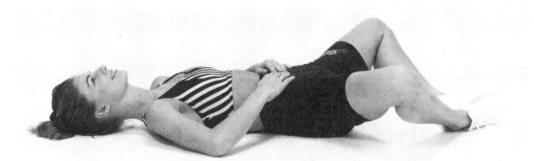

Fig 51   Lying groin stretch.

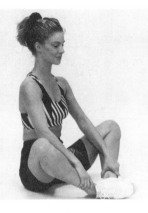

Fig 52   Seated groin stretch.

Lying Groin Stretch *(Fig 51)*

This exercise, along with the following four exercises *(Figs 52–5)*, stretches the hip adductors.

Lie flat on the floor, with your back and shoulders pressed firmly into the ground. Place the soles of your feet together and allow your knees to ease out sideways. You will feel the stretch along the insides of your thighs and groin. Breathe easily throughout the exercise.

Seated Groin Stretch *(Fig 52)*

Sit tall with good posture. Ease your legs up towards your body and place the soles of your feet together, allowing your knees to ease out down towards the floor. Make sure that your back stays long and that your shoulders are down away from your ears. Rest your hands on your lower legs or ankles, or keep them by your sides for support. You will feel the stretch along the inside of your thighs and groin. Breathe easily throughout the exercise.

If you wish to stretch the hamstrings and hip extensors at the same time, from the position above ease forward by hinging at the hip, still keeping the spine long. Breathe easily throughout the exercise *(Fig 53)*.

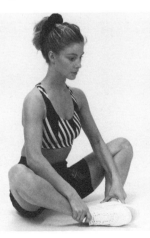

Fig 53   Seated groin stretch variation.

Standing Hurdle Stretch *(Figs 54 and 55)*

Rest one leg along the top of a high table or bar with the knee of the raised leg forward of your hips, which should also face forward. Keep your support leg extended. From this position, bend forward at the waist to reach down towards the floor. When you are comfortable, begin to flex the knee of the supporting leg. As you do so, you will feel the stretch in the inner thigh of the raised leg, as well as along the back of the support thigh and buttocks. Repeat on the other leg, breathing easily throughout the exercise.

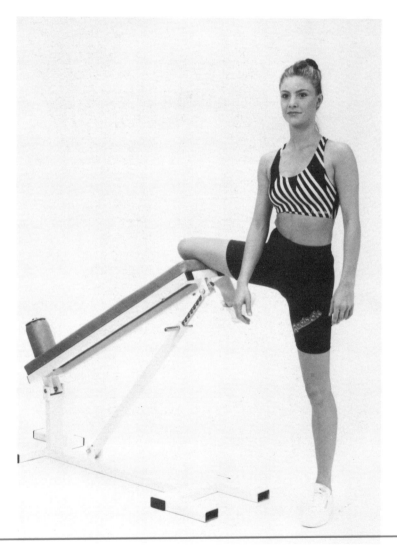

Figs 54 & 55   Standing hurdle stretch.

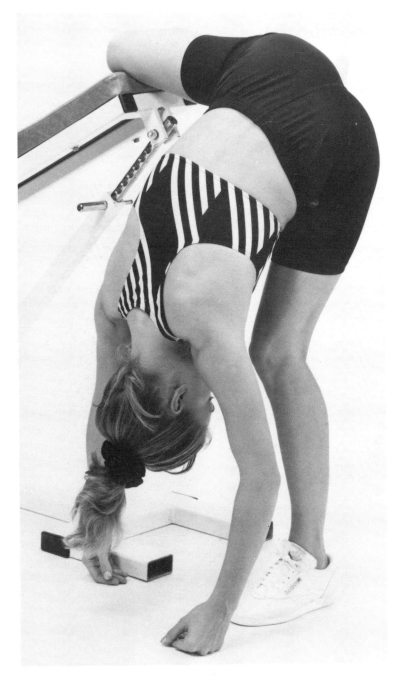

Fig 55

Seated Groin Stretch, Legs Extended (Fig 56)

Sit tall with good posture, legs outstretched and feet flexed. Make sure that your knees are pointing upwards. Use your hands for support if necessary and to help you keep your spine long. You will feel the stretch along the inner thigh and groin. Breathe easily throughout the exercise. If you can, hinge forward at the hips to increase the stretch both in the groin and in the hip extensors.

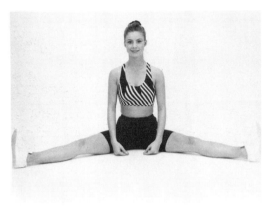

Fig 56   Seated groin stretch, legs extended.

Groin Stretch, Legs Raised (Fig 57)

The adductor muscles can also be stretched with the help of a wall. Position yourself with your buttocks as close to a wall as possible and with your back flat against the floor. Allow your heels to slide down the wall as far as possible, whilst keeping your legs extended. You will feel the stretch along the inside of your thighs and groin. Breathe easily throughout the exercise.

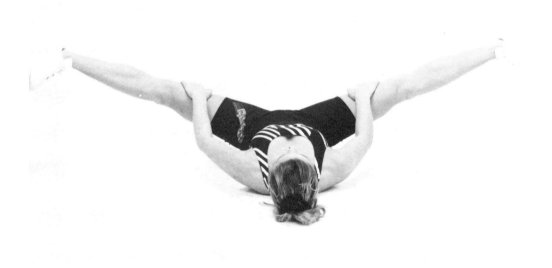

Fig 57   Groin stretch, legs raised.

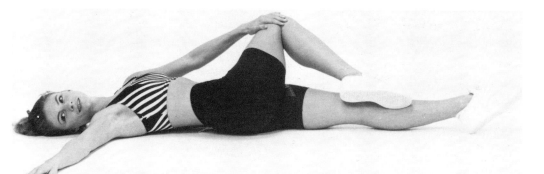

Fig 58   Lying hip abductor stretch 1.

Lying Hip Abductor Stretch 1 *(Fig 58)*

Lie flat on the floor and flex one leg up towards you whilst keeping the other leg extended. Ease the flexed leg across your extended leg, moving it further into a position of stretch with light pressure from your opposite hand. Your back and shoulders must stay in contact with the floor throughout the movement. You will feel the stretch along the outside of your hip and thigh. Breathe easily throughout the exercise.

Lying Hip Abductor Stretch 2 *(Fig 59)*

Lie flat on the floor with both legs flexed at the knee. Now cross your legs and use the weight of the top leg to bring the lower leg down towards the floor. Keep your back, shoulders and the foot of the lower leg in contact with the floor throughout the movement. You will feel the stretch along the outside of the hip and thigh. Repeat with the other leg. Breathe easily throughout the exercise.

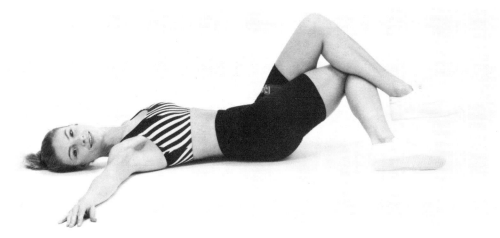

Fig 59   Lying hip abductor stretch 2.

53

No specific exercises are included for the muscles which cause either medial or lateral rotation at the hip joint, since in many of the exercises included here, rotation at the hip joint is necessary for the exercise to be performed.

STRETCHES FOR THE BACK AND TRUNK

The joints between successive vertebrae allow the spinal column to flex forwards, flex laterally (sideways), extend and rotate. The range of movement possible in each direction varies according to which part of the spinal column is involved, as discussed in Chapter 2. The muscles which cause spinal extension include the erector spinae group, gluteus maximus and trapezius. The spinal flexors (forward) include the rectus abdominis, and the internal and external oblique muscles. The lateral flexors include the obliques again and quadratus lumborum. Rotation is brought about by the obliques and a group of deep spinal rotator muscles.

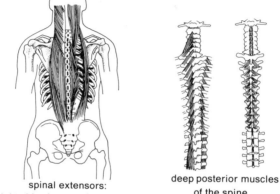

spinal extensors:
right side shows a deeper view

deep posterior muscles
of the spine

Fig 60   Muscles of the spine.

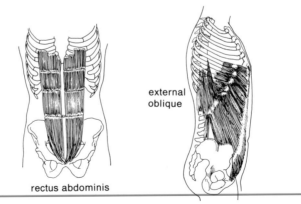

external
oblique

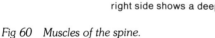
rectus abdominis

Fig 61   Muscles of the front of the trunk.

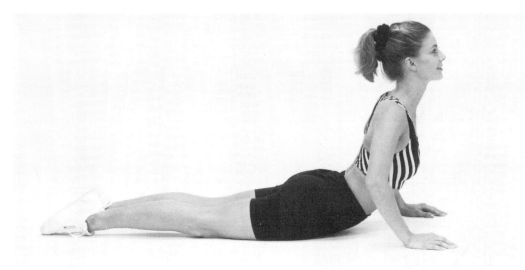

Fig 62   *Front of trunk stretch.*

Front of Trunk Stretch *(Fig 62)*

This and the next exercise *(Fig 63)* are for the forward flexors.

Lie down on the floor, fully outstretched. Slide your arms to the sides of your body for support, and ease your chest off the floor, keeping your spine long and your hips firmly pressed into the ground. You will feel the stretch in the front of the trunk. Breathe easily throughout the exercise.

Front of Trunk and Hamstring Stretch *(Fig 63)*

This is a good combination stretch which has the added advantage of strengthening and conditioning the spinal extensor muscles. Stand tall with good posture in front of a chair or table top. Flex at the knees and hips, reach forward with your arms and grasp the chair back. Now extend your spine as much as possible aiming for a straight line from hips to head. You will feel the stretch throughout the length of the front of the trunk. Breathe easily throughout. If you can, gradually straighten your legs whilst in this position, yet maintain your straight back. The long spine position is paramount in this exercise: do not sacrifice it in order to straighten your legs!

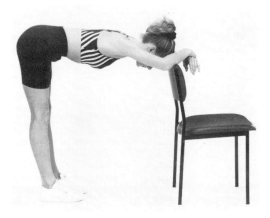

Fig 63   *Front of trunk and hamstring stretch.*

Seated Side Bend *(Fig 64)*

This exercise and the following two exercises *(Figs 66 and 67)* stretch the lateral flexors.

Sit tall with good posture on a stool or chair which has no arms. Place your hands on your hips and lift your rib-cage upwards and over to the side as far as possible, making sure your body moves sideways and not forwards or backwards. Ease as far to one side as possible and hold. You will feel the stretch along the side of the trunk opposite to the direction in which you are bending. Repeat on the other side. Breathe easily throughout the exercise.

As you become more flexible, use the extra resistance afforded by the weight of your arms to help you ease further to the side by holding them above your head as you bend to the side. Even though your arms are raised, remember to keep your shoulders down away from your ears *(see Fig 65)*.

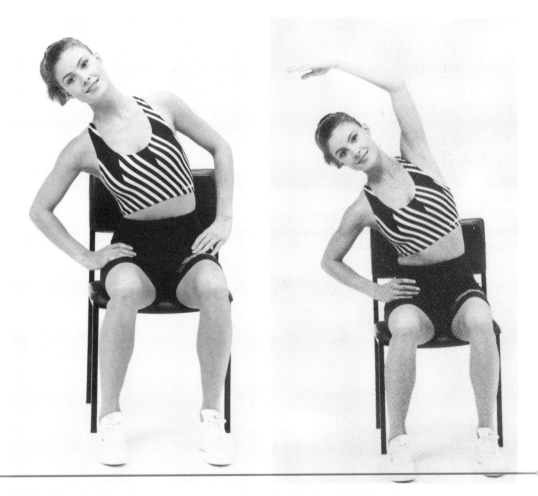

Fig 64   Seated side bend.

Fig 65   Seated side bend variation.

Standing Side Bend *(Fig 66)*

The above exercise can also be performed from the standing position. Make sure that you have a good stable base by placing your feet approximately a metre apart, toes facing forward. Bend your knees slightly and keep your hips facing forward, too. Lift up and over to the side as before, repeating on both sides.

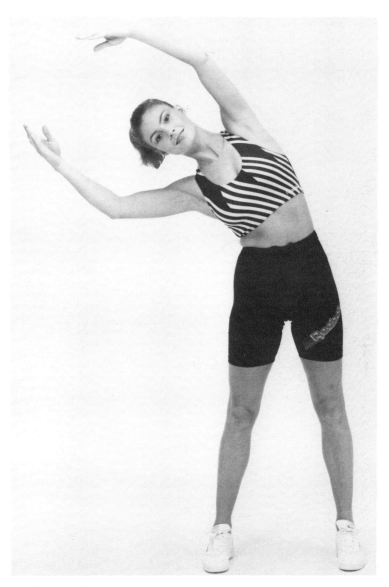

Fig 66   Standing side bend.

Sideways Neck Stretch *(Fig 67)*

Stand or sit tall with good posture, keeping your spine and neck long and your shoulders down away from your ears. Keeping your neck long, tilt your head to the side. You will feel the stretch down the side of your neck and shoulder. Repeat on the other side, breathing easily throughout. To increase the intensity of the stretch, place one hand on top of your head, using the weight of this hand to ease your head lower towards your shoulder – do not however, pull your head with this hand. *(See Fig 68)*.

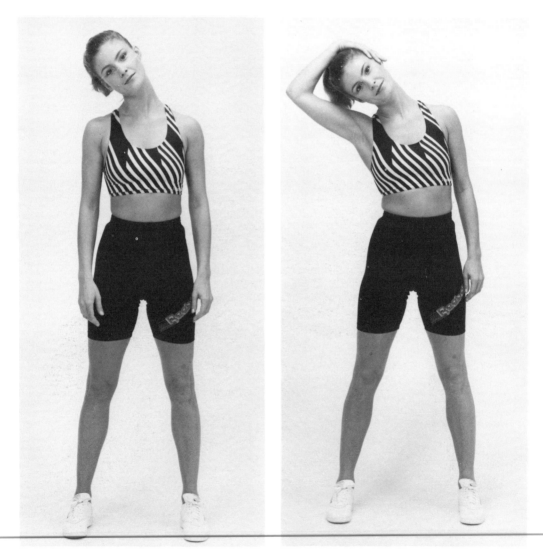

Fig 67   *Sideways neck stretch.*   Fig 68   *Sideways neck stretch variation.*

The following three exercises *(Figs 69–71)* are for the spinal extensors. Refer also to the stretches for the hamstrings and inner thigh, since many of these also involve the spinal extensor muscles.

Seated Back Release *(Fig 69)*

Sit tall with good posture and with your legs wide apart on a stool or chair which has no arms. From this position curl forwards to ease your chest between your thighs, making sure that your neck and shoulder muscles are relaxed. You will feel the stretch along the length of the back.

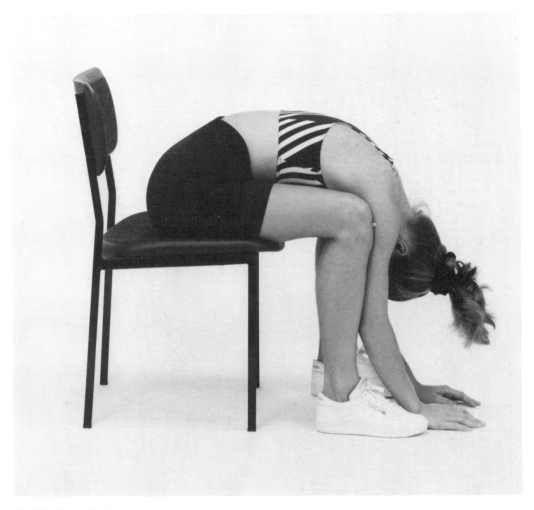

Fig 69   Seated back release.

Neck Stretch *(Fig 70)*

Stand or sit tall with good posture. Keeping your neck and spine long, shoulders down and back away from your ears, lower your chin towards your chest. You will feel the stretch along the back of your neck. Breathe easily throughout the exercise. To increase the intensity of the stretch, if you feel able, rest your hands loosely on the top of your head, allowing the weight of your upper arms to ease your head further down – do not, however, pull your head into any further position.

Diagonal Neck Stretch *(Fig 71)*

Position yourself as for the previous exercise. This time, however, turn your head to look along a diagonal, then tilt your head by bringing your chin towards your chest. You will feel the stretch along the back of your neck, shoulder and upper back. Repeat on the other side, breathing easily throughout. As before, increase the intensity of the stretch by using the weight of one hand to ease your head lower down.

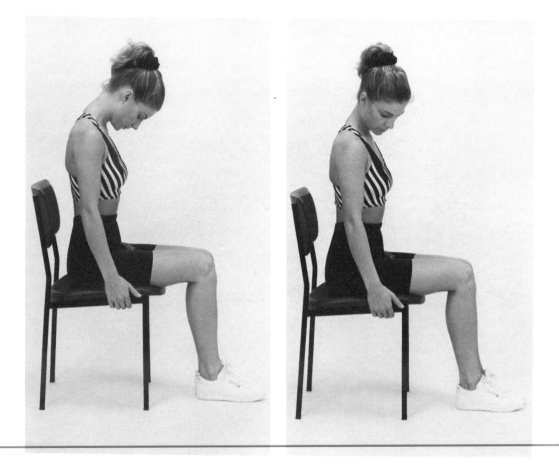

Fig 70   Neck stretch.

Fig 71   Diagonal neck stretch.

Seated Trunk Twist *(Fig 72)*

This exercise stretches the spinal rotators.

Sit tall with good posture, legs stretched out in front of you, spine long, shoulders down away from your ears. Place your right leg over your left leg as illustrated and rotate your trunk, using your left arm against your right knee to help ease you further round. Use your right arm on the floor for support. You will feel the stretch along the length of the spine as well as in the muscles around the right hip. Repeat on the opposite side, breathing easily throughout.

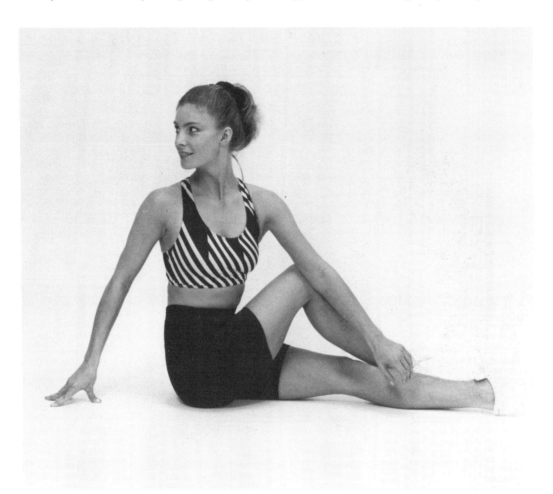

Fig 72   Seated trunk twist.

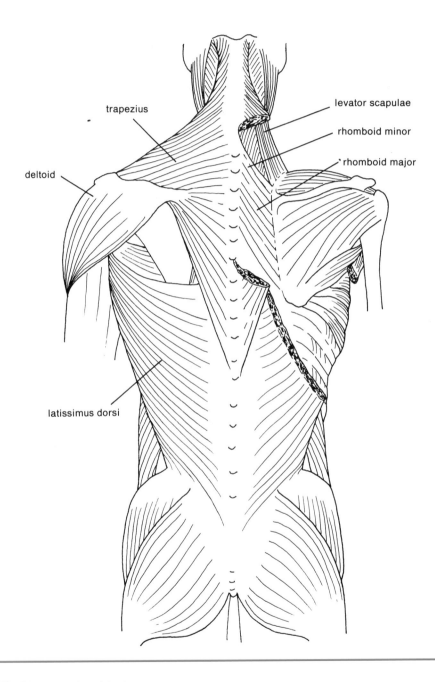

Fig 73   Major muscles of the back.

STRETCHES FOR THE MUSCLES OF THE SHOULDER GIRDLE

Four basic movements are possible at the shoulder girdle, namely elevation, depression, adduction and abduction. Muscles responsible for elevation include the trapezius and levator scapulae. Depression is also produced by the trapezius. Adduction is chiefly brought about by the trapezius and the rhomboids. Abduction is largely the job of muscles at the front of the body, such as the anterior deltoid and pectoralis major.

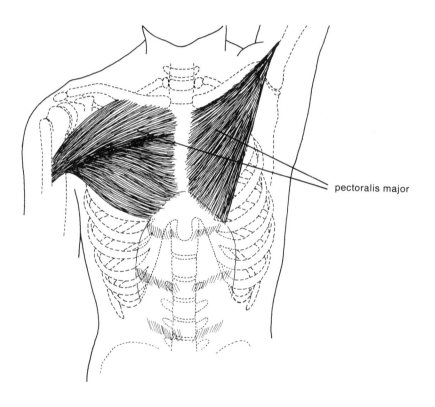

pectoralis major

Fig 74   Muscles of the chest.

Upper Back Stretch *(Fig 75)*

This exercise is an adductor stretch.

Stand or sit tall with good posture. If standing, bend your knees slightly and tilt your pelvis under. Interlock your fingers and push your hands as far away from your chest as possible, allowing your upper back to relax, whilst at the same time looking down. You will feel the stretch between your shoulder blades. Breathe easily throughout.

Chest Stretch *(Fig 76)*

This exercise is an abductor stretch.

Sit tall on a stool or stand with good posture. If standing, bend your knees slightly and tilt your pelvis under. Place your hands, loosely clasped, on the small of your back and keep your spine long and shoulders back and away from your ears. Without arching your spine, ease your elbows towards each other as far as possible, feeling the stretch in the front of the chest. Breathe easily throughout the exercise.

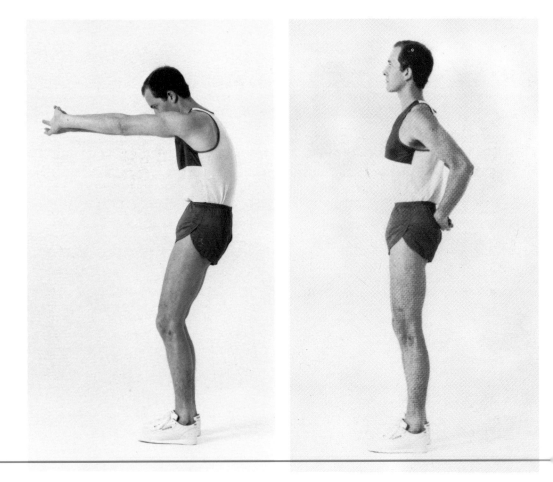

Fig 75   Upper back stretch.   *Fig 76   Chest stretch.*

STRETCHES FOR THE MUSCLES OF THE SHOULDER JOINT

The shoulder joint is a ball-and-socket joint and therefore allows the movements of flexion, extension, abduction, adduction, lateral and medial rotation, and circumduction. As with the hip joint, performing a range of exercises for flexion, extension, abduction and adduction conveniently caters for the remaining three movements. The muscles which produce flexion include the anterior deltoid and coraco-brachialis; extension is largely produced by the posterior deltoid, latissimus dorsi and teres major; adduction is produced by the latissimus dorsi and teres major; and abduction is produced by the deltoid and supraspinatus.

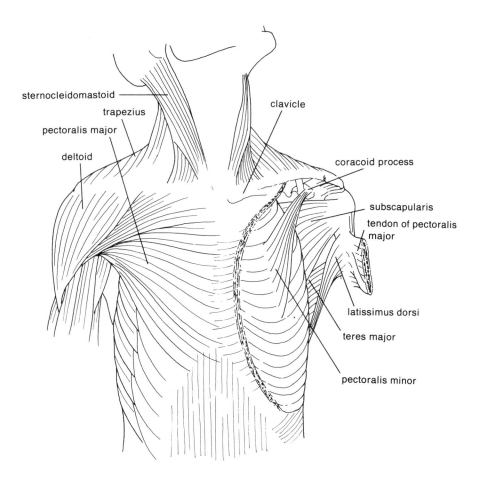

Fig 77   Muscles of the chest and shoulder.

Front of Shoulder Stretch *(Fig 78)*

This stretch is for the flexors. The chest stretch *(Fig 76)* can also be used.

Sit on a stool or stand tall with good posture. If standing, bend your knees slightly and tilt your pelvis under. Place your hands behind you, interlock your fingers and then straighten your arms and try and lift them upwards and backwards as far as possible. Keep your spine long throughout and make sure that your shoulders are back and down away from your ears. You will feel the stretch in the front of the chest. Breathe easily throughout the exercise.

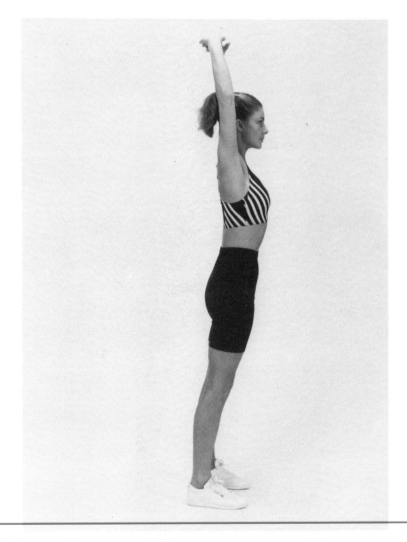

Fig 78   Front of shoulder stretch.

Shoulder and Side Stretch 1 *(Fig 79)*

The following four exercises are stretches for the extensors.

Sit on a stool or stand tall with good posture. If standing, bend your knees slightly and tilt your pelvis under. Place both hands above your head, and then place your right hand behind your left elbow, easing the left arm closer towards your head – taking the elbow behind the head if possible. Keep your spine long and your shoulders down away from your ears throughout the exercise. You will feel the stretch along the side of the trunk and shoulder. Repeat on the opposite side, breathing easily throughout.

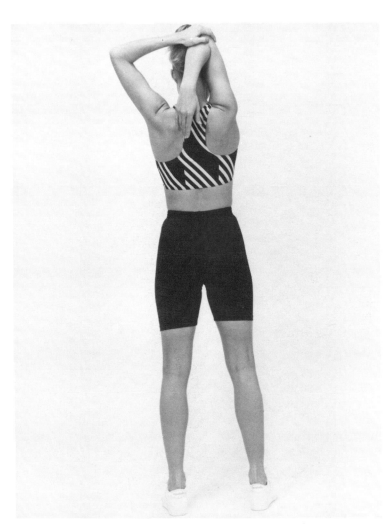

Fig 79   Shoulder and side stretch 1.

Shoulder and Side Stretch 2 *(Fig 80)*

Assume the starting position as for the previous exercise, only this time place the palms of your hands together as illustrated. Aim to straighten your arms whilst keeping your shoulders down away from your ears, feeling the stretch along the side of the trunk and shoulder. Repeat on the opposite side, breathing easily throughout the exercise.

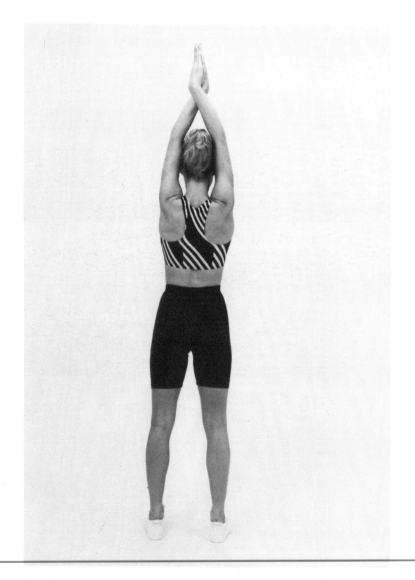

Fig 80   Shoulder and side stretch 2.

Shoulder and Side Stretch 3 *(Fig 81)*

Kneel on all fours on a mat or towel and sit back gently on your heels whilst reaching as far forward as possible with your outstretched arms. Attempt to press your buttocks and shoulders into the floor. You will feel the stretch along the side of the trunk and shoulder. Breathe easily throughout the exercise.

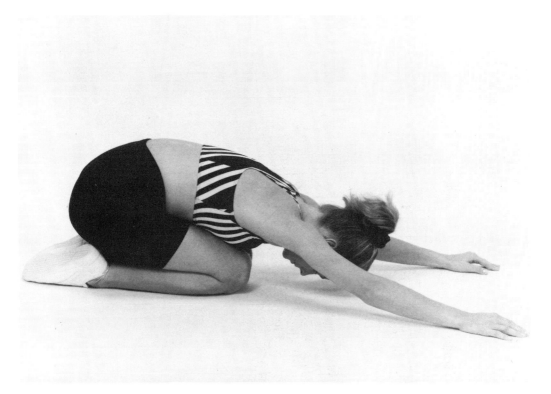

Fig 81   Shoulder and side stretch 3.

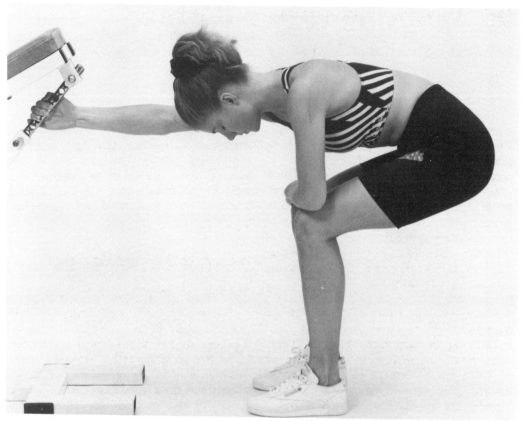

Fig 82   Side pull.

Side Pull *(Fig 82)*

Stand in front of an immovable object such as the edge of a door frame. Grasp the object firmly in one hand. Bend at the knees and hips, keep your spine long and pull against the object firmly, feeling the stretch along the side of the trunk and shoulder. Repeat on the other side, breathing easily throughout the exercise.

This list of stretches is fairly comprehensive and works all the major muscle groups of the body. You will find that the muscles of the arms (biceps, brachialis, brachioradialis and triceps) are invariably involved in the exercises for the upper back and shoulders and consequently do not have a section of their own. The same is true of the muscles of the forearms and hands. However, in this latter instance, you may like to carry out simple mobilising movements for the wrists and hands in the same way that mobilising movements for the ankle and feet were recommended *(see page 36)*.

Other stretches do, of course, exist. With the information contained in the text you should now be able to work out your own stretches and decide whether they stretch the muscles they are designed to exercise and whether they are indeed safe to perform.

5 Working with a Partner

The static stretching techniques which this book emphasises will quickly produce dramatic improvements in your range of movement. However, it is possible to employ the help of a partner to enable you to move even further into a stretch position, and to help carry out versions of PNF stretching as shown earlier in Chapter 3.

It cannot be stressed too strongly, however, that working with a partner, whilst increasing the benefit you may obtain from your stretching programme also increases the risk of injury. Any partner who is going to help you with any stretch must understand fully what they are supposed to be doing and why and must also be sympathetic to your needs and the responses of your body. If you cannot find a partner who fits this description, then do not attempt any of the following partner stretches or PNF techniques.

If you do find a suitable partner, make sure that you understand each other fully. Discuss what you are about to do and communicate throughout the movements. Above all, if a part-ner-assisted exercise is causing pain, stop doing it immediately. As with static stretching, the sensation of stretch should be mild discomfort at most. Partner stretches are best used as developmental exercises, with each stretch being held for thirty seconds.

PARTNER STRETCHES

The following short list of stretches employ a partner to help you move further into a stretch position. Once in that position, the partner maintains that position or helps you to ease further into the stretch as the sensation of stretch subsides – keep your partner informed! Throughout the exercises you should aim to be as relaxed as possible – these are not PNF exercises. Both you and your partner should read the instructions carefully before the stretch is carried out. You should breathe easily throughout all of the exercises.

Partner Back Stretch *(Fig 83)*

You should assume the kneeling position as illustrated. Your partner kneels to one side of you as shown, and places his or her left hand on the base of your spine, with the right hand towards your middle/upper back. Pressure is gently applied through both hands. The stretch should be experienced along the length of the spine.

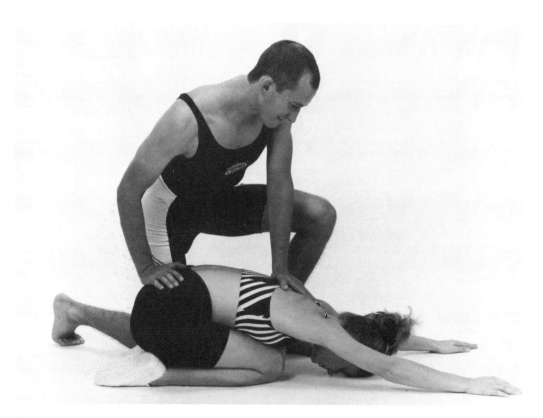

Fig 83   Partner back stretch.

Partner Groin Stretch *(Fig 84)*

Lie completely flat on the floor, with your lower back and shoulders pressed firmly into the ground. Cross your right foot over your left thigh just above the knee as shown. Your partner should position him- or herself over you as illustrated and place his or her right hand on your left hip and the left hand just above the inside of your right knee. Pressure is gently applied to both hip and knee to ease the right knee closer to the floor, whilst the left hip is kept pressed firmly into the ground. The stretch will be experienced along the inside of the crossed leg and the groin. Repeat on the opposite side.

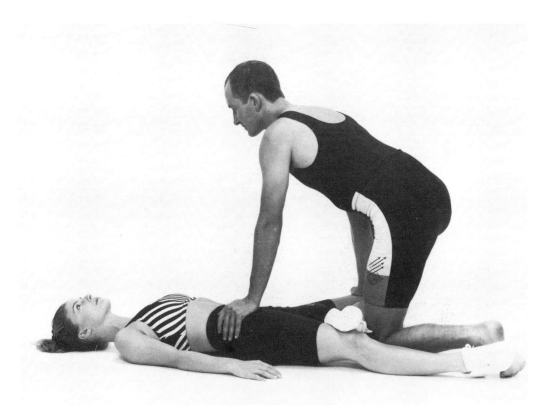

Fig 84   Partner groin stretch.

Partner Hamstring Stretch *(Fig 85)*

Lie completely flat on the floor, with your lower back and shoulders pressed firmly into the floor. Your partner sits to one side of you as shown and takes hold of your left leg at the back of the ankle and just above the knee to keep the leg fully extended. He or she gently raises the leg towards the trunk as far as possible, making sure that your hips do not leave the floor. The stretch will be experienced along the back of the raised leg. Repeat on the opposite side.

Partner Hip and Thigh Stretch *(Fig 86)*

Lie completely flat on the floor, with your lower back and shoulders pressed firmly into the floor. Your partner kneels to one side of you as illustrated and places his or her left hand on your right thigh just above the knee. The partner places his or her right hand just above the back of your left knee. Pressure is gently applied by your partner through both hands to keep your right thigh down against the floor, whilst the left thigh is eased towards your chest. The exercise is repeated on the opposite side.

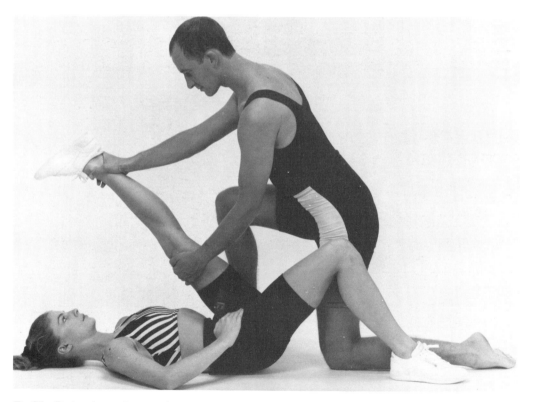

Fig 85   Partner hamstring stretch.

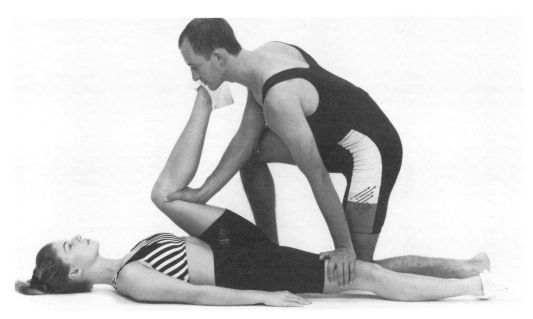

Fig 86   *Partner hip and thigh stretch.*

Partner Chest Stretch *(Fig 87)*

Sit tall with good posture on a stool or a chair with no arms. Hold both of your arms out to the side as shown. Your partner then stands directly behind you and places his or her hands around the front of your upper arms, above the elbow joint. He or she gently eases your arms backwards. You will experience the stretch across the front of your chest and shoulders. For variety, experiment with the arms at different angles above the vertical.

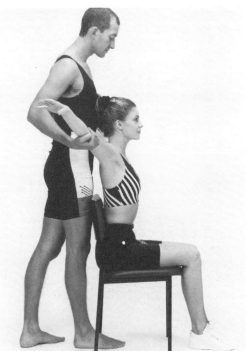

Fig 87   *Partner chest stretch.*

Obviously, there are many more partner stretches which can be carried out to help you achieve the furthermost position in each stretch. Many of the static positions illustrated in Chapter 4 can also be used with a partner. Experiment all the time, observing where the stretch is felt and comparing this to where it should be felt. Make sure in your partner work, however, that no undue stress is placed upon other joints and joint processes as the partner applies pressure. To ensure safety as much as possible, a partner should generally only apply pressure to a limb directly above or below the joints which are directly involved in the movement. This will limit the forces exerted upon other joints. For example in the last exercise given – the partner chest stretch *(Fig 87)* – note how the force is applied to the upper arms. If pressure is applied below the elbow, the force exerted on the elbow joint may cause injury.

A MODIFIED PNF TECHNIQUE

Partners are invariably necessary when performing PNF stretching exercises, although it is possible to use immovable objects in certain instances. However, if you do have the help of a knowledgeable partner, you may like to try this modified PNF technique.

In each exercise, you will be required to exert force (or push) against your partner. He or she will resist this. Each push should last for ten seconds, you should relax fully whilst your partner eases your limb further into the stretch position for a further ten seconds. This process should be repeated three times – push for ten seconds, ease for ten seconds, push for ten seconds and so on.

As with the previous sequence of partner stretches, both subject and partner should read all the instructions for each exercise carefully before attempting any of the stretches.

PNF Partner Hamstring Stretch *(Fig 88)*

Assume the position as in the partner hamstring stretch *(Fig 85)*. Your partner should also assume the position as described in that exercise. He or she should ask your subject to press firmly against his or her right hand for ten seconds by strongly contracting your hamstring muscles. The partner resists this movement through firm pressure so that your leg does not move. After ten seconds, your partner instructs you to relax completely and then tries to ease your leg closer towards your chest until a furthermost position is reached and holds this for ten seconds. From this new position, your partner instructs you to push against him or her again, repeating the process a total of three times. The same sequence of movements is then performed on the opposite leg.

PNF Partner Hip and Thigh Stretch *(Fig 89)*

You and your partner should assume the positions described in the partner hip and thigh stretch *(Fig 86)*. Your partner asks you to push against both of his or her hands for ten seconds. He or she resists this movement through firm pressure so that neither of your legs move. After ten seconds, your partner instructs you to relax completely and tries to ease your raised leg closer to your thigh, whilst easing your extended leg flat against the floor. Your partner should ensure that your spine does not arch, but stays in contact with the floor at all times. Having reached a new furthermost position, your partner instructs you to push against his or her hands again, and you repeat the sequence as before a total of three times. The exercise is repeated on the opposite leg.

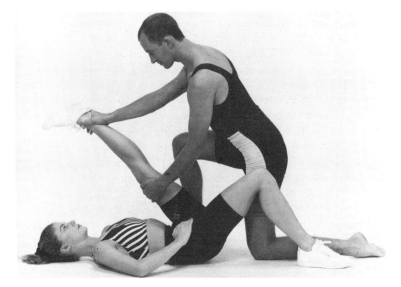

Fig 88   PNF partner hamstring stretch.

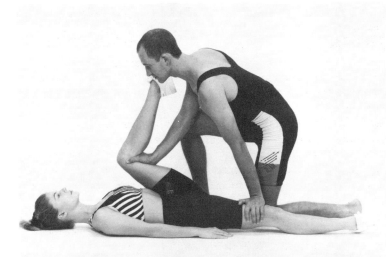

Fig 89   PNF partner hip and thigh stretch.

PNF Partner Groin Stretch *(Fig 90)*

Lie flat with your hips, shoulders and spine pressed firmly into the floor. Bend your knees to approximately right angles, place the soles of your feet together and allow your knees to ease out to the side. Your partner kneels in front of you and places his or her hands on the inside of your thighs just above your knees. He or she instructs you to press against his or her hands to try and move your knees upwards for ten seconds. Your partner should resist this movement so that your knees do not move. After ten seconds, your partner instructs you to relax completely and then tries to ease your knees closer to the floor by gently applying pressure through his or her hands. After ten seconds, repeat. Perform the whole sequence a total of three times.

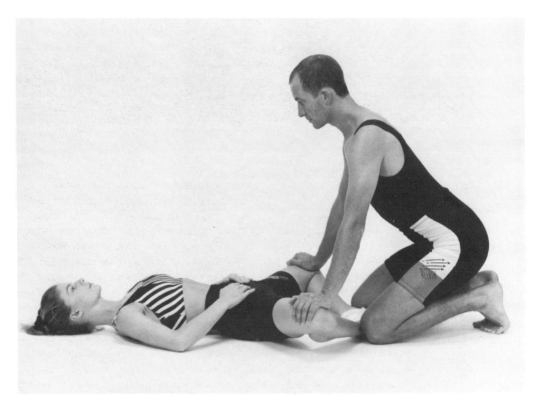

Fig 90   PNF partner groin stretch.

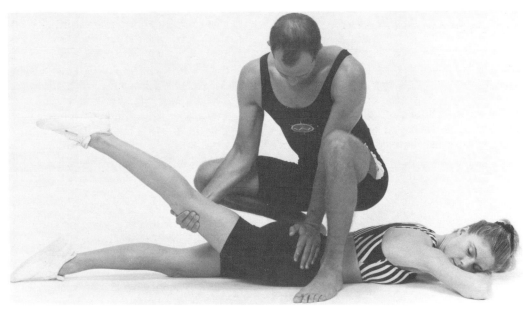

Fig 91   PNF partner hip flexor stretch.

PNF Partner Hip Flexor Stretch *(Fig 91)*

Lie face down with your hips and shoulders pressed firmly into the floor. Your partner squats over you as illustrated, pressing his or her left hand firmly against your right hip and holding your right leg under the front of your right thigh with his or her right hand, so that it is off the floor as much as possible. Your partner instructs you to press against his or her right hand whilst he or she resists this movement for ten seconds. Your partner then asks you to relax completely, whilst he or she tries to ease your thigh further towards him or her without letting your hips come off the floor. After ten seconds, repeat. Perform the whole sequence a total of three times with each leg.

PNF Chest Stretch

Both you and your partner assume the positions described in the partner chest stretch *(Fig 87)*.

He or she instructs you to push against his or her hands to try and bring your arms forward for ten seconds. Your partner resists this movement and after ten seconds instructs you to relax as he or she eases your arms further backwards for ten seconds, ensuring that your spine stays long throughout the movement. Repeat the sequence three times.

These are just a representative sample of how you might introduce a modified PNF technique easily and safely into your stretching programmes. As with the partner exercises given earlier, it is worthwhile experimenting with other exercises to see whether they lend themselves to the same simple modified technique. You must, however, be careful! – your partner should listen to you carefully and you should both discuss each stretch and exercise position before you attempt it.

6 Improving Your Posture

In Chapter 1 it was pointed out that poor posture, whether sitting or standing, is related to a host of minor injuries and problems. Poor posture also does little for your overall appearance. It has further been observed that any exercising done with poor posture invariably leads to injury.

People exhibiting perfect posture are rare since poor posture can be caused in so many ways. Essentially there are seven major factors to be considered when trying to find the cause or causes of an individual's bad posture. Injury, for example, can be a major postural problem since many injuries will actually weaken the structure and framework of the body, consequently throwing it out of balance. This is also true of certain diseases, which may again weaken muscles and joints. Apart from keeping as healthy as possible and following the correct rehabilitation programme following any kind of traumatic injury, there is very little that can be done about these two causes of improper posture.

There is also little that can easily be done if poor posture is inherited as in the case of lateral curvature of the spine (scoliosis). Invariably, scoliosis needs specialist treatment and even surgery if lateral curvature is excessive. Many experts also agree that there are emotional aspects of poor posture which need to be considered – how a person stands, sits and moves may well reflect his or her emotional status. Again, specialist treatment will be necessary in such instances. There are, however, several aspects of poor posture which can be dealt with quite easily by the individual. These are imbalances in the strength and muscular endurance of various muscle groups, improper attire and bad habits.

Taking bad habits first, ask yourself how often have you found yourself slumping over a desk, slouching in a chair, or standing in a 'twisted' position. Do you always carry a bag over the same shoulder, or a briefcase in the same hand? The positions which you place your body in during everyday situations are arguably the single most important cause of poor posture in the majority of people. Habitually carrying out these activities with poor posture invariably leads to the shortening of various muscles which in turn leads to an improper relationship between the various segments of the body. Similarly, wearing high-heeled shoes on a regular basis leads to excessive shortening of the muscles of the back of the calf and wearing tight clothing leads to restricted joint movements. The end results are the same – a loss of normal joint mobility which in turn leads to poor posture.

In many instances individuals having muscles groups which are much stronger or weaker than others means that certain movements or actions occur far more readily in one direction than in the other direction. Possessing weak abdominal muscles and strong, short hip flexor and back muscles often causes the pelvis to tilt leading to an exaggerated curvature of the spine known as lumbar lordosis. 'Round' shoulders are often a result of the individual having short, strong muscles at the front of the chest, and weak shoulder girdle adductor muscles. In these instances and others improving joint mobility and balancing out the relative strengths of muscles will lead to dramatic improvements in your general posture and appearance.

POSTURE IMPROVEMENT PLAN

1   Check your initial posture – you will need a mirror and the help of a friend for this. Compare your posture as carefully as possible to the good standing posture shown in *Fig 99*. Note the relative positioning of your body parts compared to the diagrams. Is one shoulder higher than the other, for example? Are your hips even? Is your spine curved excessively in any direction? Does your head poke forward? Make a note of any obvious deviations from the ideal postural positions shown.

2   *Figs 92, 94 and 96* indicate three common problem postures. Do any of them apply to you? If they do, refer to the Posture Programme tables.

3   Try to improve your sitting, standing and moving habits. A good sitting posture is indicated in *Fig 98*. Good standing posture is shown in *Fig 99* and good walking posture is shown in *Fig 100*. If you find yourself sitting for a considerable length of time whether at work or home, carry out the short sequence of sitting stretches given in Stretching Programme 2. Good posture and technique for lifting and carrying are given in *Fig 101*.

4   Try not to wear restrictive clothing or shoes whenever possible. If you can, take off your shoes at work or when seated in the home as this will allow you to carry out the foot and toe mobility exercises given on page 36 whenever you feel the urge. Also, always stretch your calves if you have been wearing high heels for any length of time.

5   Carry out the General Stretching Programme given on page 88, or one similar at least every other day.

COMMON POSTURE PROBLEMS

Lordosis *(Fig 92)*

In the position of lumbar lordosis illustrated, the excessive curvature of the spine is the result of a lack of flexibility and a shortening of the spinal extensor muscles in the lower back and also of the hip flexor muscles. Invariably the abdominal muscles are weak. Follow Posture Programme 1 *(Fig 93)*, as well as the General Stretching Programme *(Fig 106)*.

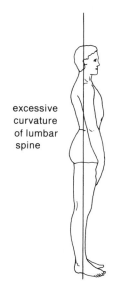

excessive
curvature
of lumbar
spine

Fig 92   Lordosis.

POSTURE PROGRAMME 1

Kneeling hip flexor stretch	*(Fig 49)*
Seated hamstring/lower back stretch	*(Fig 42)*
Abdominal curl	*(Figs 102 & 103)*
Abdominal crunch	*(Figs 104 & 105)*

Hold each stretch for thirty seconds and repeat the programme three times.

Fig 93

Flat Back *(Fig 94)*

Whilst there are many variations of muscle short-ness and inflexibility in this posture it is usually a result of tight hamstrings. Follow Posture Pro-gramme 2 *(Fig 95)*, as well as the General Stretching Programme.

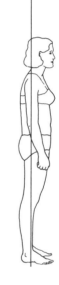

Fig 94   Flat back posture.

POSTURE PROGRAMME 2

Lying hamstring stretch	*(Fig 38)*
Abdominal curl	*(Figs 102 & 103)*
Abdominal crunch	*(Figs 104 & 105)*

Hold each stretch for thirty seconds and repeat the programme three times.

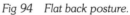

Fig 95

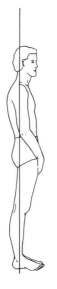

Fig 96   Sway back posture.

Sway Back *(Fig 96)*

In this posture, the muscles which generally need stretching include the hamstrings and lower back muscles and the muscles in the front of the chest. Follow Posture Programme 3 *(Fig 97)*, as well as the General Stretching Programme.

POSTURE PROGRAMME 3

Lying hamstring stretch	*(Fig 38)*
Chest stretch	*(Fig 76)*
Abdominal curl	*(Figs 102 & 103)*
Abdominal crunch	*(Figs 104 & 105)*

Hold each stretch for thirty seconds and repeat the programme three times.

Fig 97

ACQUIRING GOOD POSTURE

Good Sitting Posture *(Fig 98)*

When sitting, aim to sit tall in your chair so that the spine is fully lengthened whilst maintaining its natural curves. You should feel that the bones of your spinal column are stacked neatly on top of one another. Aim to keep your shoulders down and back. Have your hips facing forwards and your feet flat on the floor if possible. Do not allow your tummy to 'sag' forward. Bear this good sitting posture in mind whether sitting at a desk, table, in the car, or when watching television.

Good Standing Posture *(Fig 99)*

As with sitting, stand tall, have your hips facing forwards, pelvis 'centred' and your legs straight, but not locked at the knee. Keep your feet a comfortable distance apart so that you feel stable and relaxed. Avoid the tendency to slouch or stand so that all of your weight is concentrated on one leg. Keep your feet flat on the floor so that your weight is spread evenly and not directed through either the inside or outside of your feet.

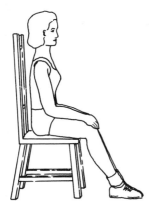

Fig 98   Good sitting posture.

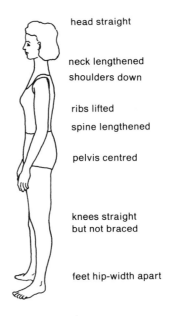

head straight

neck lengthened
shoulders down

ribs lifted
spine lengthened

pelvis centred

knees straight
but not braced

feet hip-width apart

Fig 99   Good standing posture.

Good Walking Posture *(Fig 100)*

Always aim to walk tall. You should also push off firmly from your back leg with each stride and get a full range of movement at the hip joint. Your arms should swing loosely by your sides.

Good Lifting And Carrying Posture *(Fig 101)*

The golden rules for lifting and carrying objects are simple. Firstly, always ensure that you are as close as possible to the object to be lifted or moved. Then, make sure that you use the strongest muscles available for the task: these are the large muscles around the hips and thighs. Effectively all the effort comes from the legs, whilst the spine is kept long – *Fig 101* illustrates this.

When carrying objects, try and keep the object close to your body and if possible, even up the weight so that an equal amount of work is done by both sides of the body. It is far better in terms of your posture to carry two light bags (one in each hand) than one heavy bag. If you do carry just one bag, try and swap hands on a regular basis so that both sides of your body are stressed equally.

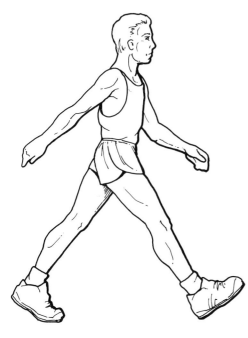

Fig 100   Good walking posture.

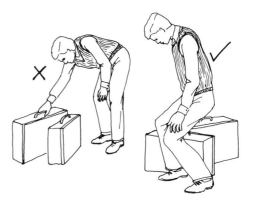

Fig 101   Good lifting and carrying posture.

STRENGTHENING EXERCISES FOR THE ABDOMINAL MUSCLES

Abdominal Curl (Figs 102 and 103)

Lie flat on the floor with your knees bent at an angle of approximately ninety degrees. Have your arms resting loosely by your sides or fold them across your chest. Making sure that your lower back is pressed firmly on to the floor at all times, smoothly curl your head and shoulders off the floor to ease further towards your thighs. The fitter you become, the closer to your thighs you will be able to go. Having reached your uppermost position, slowly curl down and repeat the curl up as soon as your mid-back touches the floor. Breathe out as you curl up, and breathe in as you curl down.

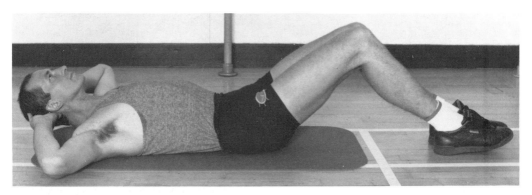

Figs 102 & 103   Abdominal curl.

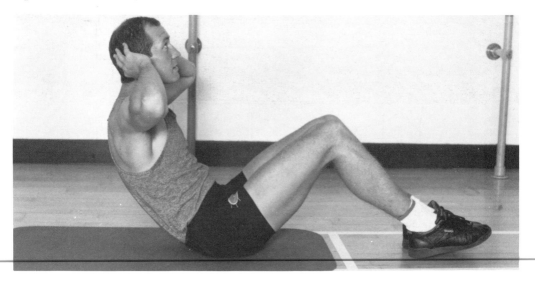

Fig 103

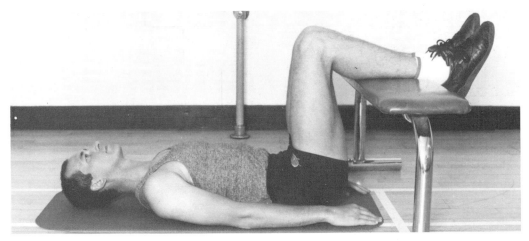

Figs 104 & 105   Abdominal crunch.

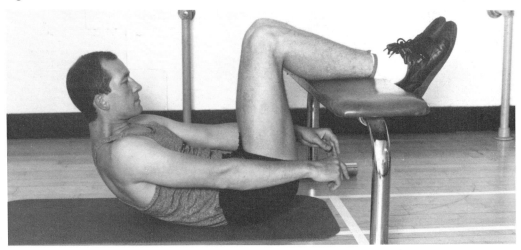

Fig 105

Abdominal Crunch (Figs 104 and 105)

Lie flat on the floor with your lower legs resting on a bench or chair so that your knees are directly above your hips. Now try and perform the curl up as before, holding your uppermost position momentarily before curling down. Repeat, breathing out as you curl up and breathing in as you curl down.

With both of these exercises, try and perform them with a smooth, regular rhythm aiming to carry out twelve complete repetitions in each case. As you become fitter, increase the number of repetitions gradually until you can perform thirty of each exercise. Never sacrifice exercise technique in order to perform more repetitions.

7 Sports Specific Programmes

The benefits of regular stretching as far as sportsmen and women are concerned have been fully outlined in Chapter 1. All sports performers will experience an improvement in their training and performance as their mobility and flexibility improves. The General Stretching Programme given below may be used by all performers, either as a preparatory stretching routine prior to training or, if the stretches are held for longer, as a developmental routine. Additional exercises for specific sports are given under the appropriate heading.

Remember: preparatory stretches need only be held for six seconds; developmental stretches need to be held for thirty seconds.

GENERAL STRETCHING PROGRAMME

Warm-up

Standing calf stretch (gastrocnemius)	(Fig 23)
Standing calf stretch (soleus)	(Fig 25)
Front of lower leg stretch	(Fig 28)
Standing quadriceps stretch	(Fig 34)
Standing hamstring stretch	(Figs 36 & 37)
Kneeling hip flexor stretch	(Fig 49)
Lying groin stretch	(Fig 51)
Lying hip abductor stretch 1	(Fig 58)
Standing side bend	(Fig 66)
Sideways neck stretch	(Fig 67)
Neck stretch	(Fig 70)
Upper back stretch	(Fig 75)
Chest stretch	(Fig 76)

Fig 106

General Stretching Programme *(Fig 106)*

A general stretching programme should aim to include exercises for all the major muscle groups in the body. The programme given in *Fig 106* is only an example. It is quite possible to substitute any exercise for another exercise for the same body part if you wish. You may use the simple warm-up given earlier in Chapter 4 or you may like to structure your own warm-up sequence using the guide-lines given in the same chapter. Naturally, you may add any extra exercises to the sequence given if you wish or substitute favourite exercises of your own. Work through the exercises smoothly.

Seated Stretching Programme *(Fig 107)*

For anyone who is desk-bound for any length of time, the programme given in *Fig 107* can be performed whilst seated and may come in useful. Ideally you should try to warm up thoroughly before carrying out this programme. This is obviously not possible if you are in a busy office, so ease into each stretch position with more caution than you would do normally.

SEATED STRETCHING PROGRAMME	
Seated side bend	*(Fig 64)*
Upper back stretch	*(Fig 75)*
Chest stretch	*(Fig 76)*
Front of shoulder stretch	*(Fig 78)*
Shoulder and side stretch 1	*(Fig 79)*
Neck stretch	*(Fig 70)*
Sideways neck stretch	*(Fig 67)*
Foot circling	*(Fig 29)*
Invert and evert feet	*(Fig 30)*
Flex and extend toes	*(Fig 31)*
Toe spread	*(Fig 32)*

Fig 107

Runners' Stretching Programme (Fig 108)

Running involves all the muscles of the lower body and many of those of the trunk and upper body. The range of movement at each joint when running largely depends upon the speed at which the runner is travelling: the faster he or she moves, the greater the range of movement. It could therefore be argued that sprinters should spend more time engaged in warming up and preparatory stretching than the average jogger, though this is not to say that a jogger will derive any less benefit from a stretching programme.

If there are specific weaknesses in your technique that you are aware of which you think may be helped by any of the stretching exercises listed in this book, then include them in your programme.

RUNNERS' STRETCHING PROGRAMME

A good general warm-up should be followed by a good stretching programme plus:

Foot circling	(Fig 29)
Invert and evert feet	(Fig 30)
Flex and extend toes	(Fig 31)
Toe spread	(Fig 32)

More exercises should also be included for the hamstrings and the groin, such as:

Seated groin stretch variation	(Fig 53)
Seated hamstring/lower back stretch	(Fig 42)

More work for the hip flexors is also a good idea, for example:

Lying hip flexor stretch	(Fig 50)

Fig 108

Cyclists' Stretching Programme *(Fig 109)*

Cyclists are probably well-advised to follow a similar programme to that advocated for the runners. In addition, they may like to include more back and quadriceps exercises such as those given in *Fig 109*.

Rowers' Stretching Programme

Rowers may like to follow a similar programme to that given for cyclists, again paying specific attention to the upper back and trunk muscles.

CYCLISTS' STRETCHING PROGRAMME

Follow the Runners' Stretching Programme (*Fig 108*) plus the following exercises:

Lying quadriceps stretch	(*Fig 35*)
Front of trunk and hamstring stretch	(*Fig 63*)
Seated trunk twist	(*Fig 72*)
Side pull	(*Fig 82*)

Fig 109

Swimmers' Stretching Programme *(Fig 110)*

Swimmers should consult the runners' routine (*Fig 108*), as well as including more exercises for the shoulders and shoulder girdle muscles such as those given in *Fig 110*.

Racket Players' Stretching Programme

Follow the General Stretching Programme (*Fig 106*), adding the extra upper body stretches as advocated for swimmers, plus the additional hamstring and groin exercises for runners.

SWIMMERS' STRETCHING PROGRAMME

Consult the Runners' Stretching Programme (*Fig 108*) plus the following exercises:

Shoulder and side stretch 1	(*Fig 79*)
Side pull	(*Fig 82*)
Partner chest stretch	(*Fig 87*)

Fig 110

Designing Any Sports Stretching Programme

The above programmes should illustrate quite clearly how to put your stretching programme together whatever your sport. Centre your programme around a general sequence of exercises, then add extra exercises for the muscle groups which are most involved in the sports activity itself. You should also include exercises which are necessary as far as your personal technique is concerned.

Further Reading

Fox, E. L. and Matthews, D. K. *The Physiological Basis of Physical Education and Athletics* (Saunders, 1981).

Francis, P. and Francis, L. *If It Hurts, Don't Do It* (Prima, 1988).

Holt, L. E. *et al* 'A comparative study of three stretching techniques', *Perceptual and Motor Skills*, 31 (1970), 611–16.

Kendall, P. F. and Kendall, McCreary E. *Muscles, Testing and Function* (Williams & Wilkins, 1983).

MacDougall, J. D., Wenger, H. A. and Green, H. J. *Physiological Testing of the Elite Athlete* (Mouvement Publications, 1982).

National Strength Conditioning Association 'Flexibility', *NSCA Journal*, August–September (1984), 10–22, 71–3.

Prentice, W. E. 'A comparison of static stretching and PNF stretching for improving hip joint flexibility', *Athletic Training*, 18 (1983), 56–9.

Wells, K. F. and Luttgens, K. *Kinesiology* (Saunders, 1976).

Index